# LOOKING GOOD

### Sally Ann Voak

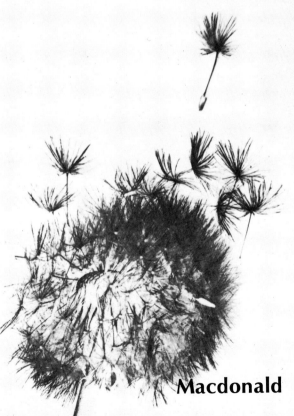

**Macdonald**

**Editorial manager**
Chester Fisher
**Series editor**
Jim Miles
**Editor**
Linda Sonntag
**Picture research**
Anne Williams
**Production**
Penny Kitchenham

Published in association with
Thames Television's programme
*After Noon*, produced by
Catherine Freeman

First published 1978
Macdonald Educational Ltd
Holywell House
Worship Street
London EC2A 2EN

Made and printed by
Waterlow (Dunstable) Ltd

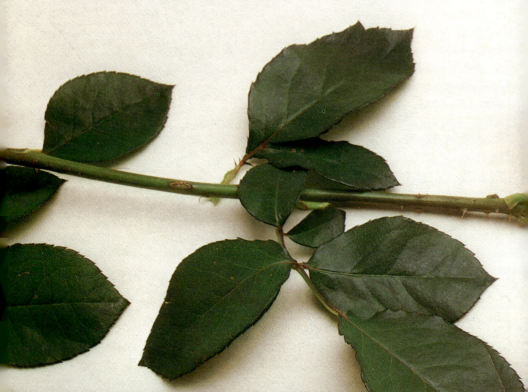

# Contents

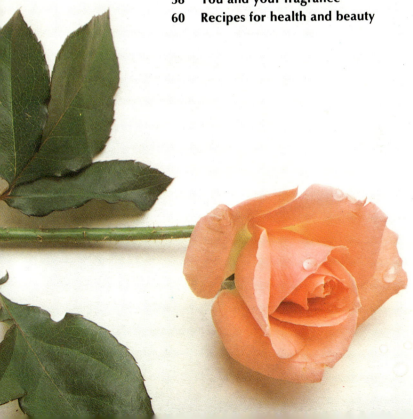

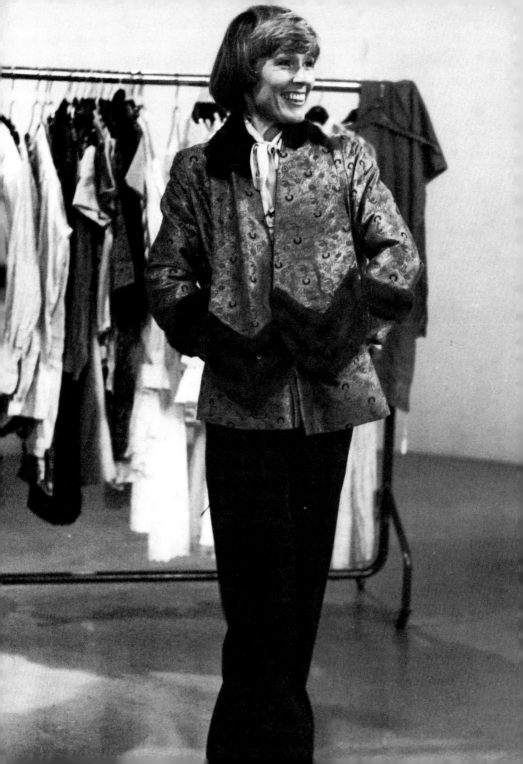

# Introduction

The Thames Television 'After Noon' programmes treat the subject of beauty in a positive, realistic way. So does this book. It aims, like the programmes, to help you make the most of your good points, to clarify the often-confusing ideas that surround the beauty business and to help you plan a simple, effective routine for a lifetime of healthy, natural good looks.

Included are many of the ideas of tall, attractive Mary Parkinson, the presenter of the programmes which cover style and beauty. Mary, who's a busy mother as well as a successful career woman, believes that everyone can improve their looks—but they must start with two important basics: good health and a sense of humour! 'I'm a strong advocate of healthy eating', she says, 'but I don't believe in sacrificing everything for a reed-slim shape. I think enjoying life—including food—is a vital part of looking great. I also feel that no-one should become boringly obsessive about beauty. It should be fun—not a chore.'

To make beauty fun (and practical, too), 'Looking Good' includes all the latest, brightest, and simplest beauty tricks, plus the fascinating scientific information that backs up these new ideas.

◀ Mary Parkinson, presenter of the 'After Noon' beauty programmes.

# Your body is a beauty machine

The very first essential of looking good is to eat well. Eating 'well' doesn't mean that you should gorge yourself, but that you should be selective about food, and make sure that you eat and drink the things that will help your skin, hair, teeth, eyes and body generally to stay in top form.

The body really does act as a kind of machine, efficiently using nutrients (vitamins, minerals, proteins, carbohydrates, fats, trace elements and roughage) from food to rebuild and nourish tissues and cells. If your diet lacked sufficient quantities of these nutrients, you would eventually become ill, and nutritionists are aware that many people do experience symptoms of undernourishment, even in our affluent society. They call these symptoms 'clinical food deficiency': they are not bad enough to need medical attention, but do cause certain problems such as tiredness, spots, dry skin, dull hair, brittle nails and even bad breath.

The illustration opposite shows which vitamins and minerals are needed for specific beauty areas, and in which foods these are found. You also need:

*Protein* (in meat, fish, eggs, cheese, soya beans, nuts, lentils) is the body-building nutrient. Skin, hair, nails, all need protein, particularly for repair and growth, and your diet should include some every day.

*Fats* (in animal foods like milk, cheese, meat and vegetable foods like vegetable oils and fish oils) supply energy and carry nutrients, such as vitamin A and vitamin D in fish oils. They also make other foods more palatable: a total lack of fat in a diet would result in a pretty unappetising menu! However, evidence that animal fats are a contributory factor in heart disease has made many people switch to vegetable fats, which is fine, if your doctor advises this. If not, this could result in a depletion of vitamins and minerals. So it's essential to check before you go on a low-fat diet.

*Carbohydrates* (in bread, potatoes, root vegetables, pasta, rice, sweet foods) supply energy. They also supply around half the calories in most people's diets. Foods like hamburger buns, crisps, chocolate, sweets, sweet drinks and snacks are certainly good for pushing up your blood-sugar level and giving instant satisfaction. If you are in a heavy manual job, they are vital. However, they do have a disadvantage from a beauty point of view. That quick 'lift' is almost always followed by a 'low', and a craving for more carbohydrate foods. Since these foods do put on weight and, in the case of sugary foods, often supply few other nutrients, they are dangerous for your looks. The exception? Bread, which, if it is wholemeal, supplies such useful amounts of the 'B' vitamins, roughage, vitamin E and trace minerals that it is a vital part of your beauty diet. Potatoes, too, are rich in vitamin C, unless overcooked, and contain trace minerals and roughage in the skins, so they do work for your beauty plan.

*Roughage* is the name given to the fibrous parts of foods which surround the nutrients. Although it is not in itself a contributor to the cell renewal and body-building processes, it does help food pass through the body rapidly and efficiently. There are also indications that roughage helps prevent serious diseases like diverticulitis (small 'blowouts' in the colon), bowel cancer and haemorrhoids (commonly known as piles).

## Clear skin
Vitamins B2, B6; niacin (yeast, wheatgerm, liver, kidney); vitamin C (citrus fruits); protein (meat, fish, eggs, cheese).

## Healthy teeth
Calcium (milk, cheese, parsley, yogurt); fluorine (in drinking water in certain areas, seafoods, tea); zinc (oysters, liver, sweetbreads).

## Glossy hair
Protein (meat, fish, eggs, cheese); iron (liver, red meat, egg yolk, lentils, watercress).

## Shining eyes
Vitamin A (fish liver oils, liver, eggs, yogurt, butter, green vegetables, carrots); vitamin C (citrus fruits); zinc (oysters, liver, sweetbreads).

## Strong fingernails
Protein (meat, fish, eggs, cheese); calcium (milk, cheese, parsley, yogurt); phosphorus (milk, cheese, egg yolk, wholemeal flour, nuts, meat).

## Strong bones and muscles
Calcium (milk, cheese, parsley, yogurt); protein (meat, fish, eggs, cheese); phosphorus (milk, cheese, egg yolk, wholemeal flour, nuts, meat). Sulphur (nuts, dried fruit, oatmeal, barley); vitamin D, especially necessary during pregnancy, (fish liver oils, eggs, milk, butter, sunshine on skin).

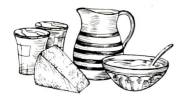

Dairy foods contain protein, vitamin A, vitamin D, and fat. An excellent source of calcium and phosphorus.

Vital during pregnancy, protein is the body-building nutrient milk a natural tranquillizer. A are good for skin and teeth.

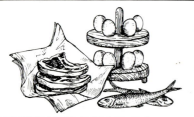

Eggs, red meat and offal contain iron and the B group of vitamins, copper, manganese and zinc. Fish contains iodine and sodium.

Essential for healthy skin, nails, hair, eyes, sex life, and for correct balance of nervous energy and body fluids.

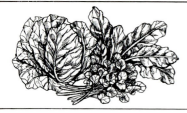

Leafy vegetables contain vitamin C, which is easily destroyed by overcooking, roughage, folic acid, vitamin K and iron.

Give a clear and healthy skin and a natural resistance to infection. Top up your supply when colds are around, especially if you smoke.

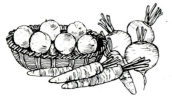

All these contain carotene, a yellow pigment, which the body uses to manufacture vitamin A, and roughage.

Carotene is necessary for healthy eyes and you need more if you work under fluorescent lights.

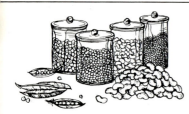

Pulses are high in protein and a good substitute for meat or fish. They also contain sodium, potassium, magnesium, sulphur.

Body-building, highly nutritious foods which are high in calories: so slimmers should limit them.

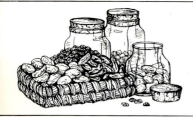

Dried fruits are sources of sulphur, sodium and potassium.

Sulphur helps construct body cells. Sodium and potassium jointly help the body's fluid balance.

Sufficient roughage also prevents constipation, and although this is not a disease, it's hard to feel beautiful if you're constipated.

Unfortunately, food processing often destroys dietary fibre. The best sources are the natural foods: fruit, with skins, whole cereals and grains such as bran, fresh vegetables, brown rice and pasta, beans and lentils. Sufficient roughage in the diet also helps to keep you slim, since it makes you feel satisfied. It's possible to preserve roughage very simply in cooking by always cooking vegetables in their skins, for a short while only, adding bran to cereals and puddings and serving raw foods at each meal.

## An apple a day

Here are some simple rules for your everyday eating pattern:
1. Eat fresh fruit and lightly-cooked vegetables such as greens or carrots *every single day*. Leave the skins on where possible.
2. Eat a protein food from a fish, vegetable and animal source *every three days*. You could have cod or herrings one day, lentil hot-pot the next, then stew or cauliflower cheese the next to ensure that you get protein from different sources. You do *not* need meat every single day.
3. Eat some fresh nuts and liver or kidney *every week*.
Drink milk alone or in tea or coffee and plenty of water. If you can afford to, drink a glass or two of red wine *each day* to relax and calm you and to add extra iron to your diet. Choose fresh, unsweetened fruit and vegetable juices and avoid high-carbohydrate squashes and soft drinks.

## Natural pick-me-ups

Because of our ghastly dietary habits, we frequently miss out on vital nutrients. Many women go short of iron during and just after menstruation, and feel below par and droopy as a result. Egg yolk, liver, meat, watercress and lentils are all good sources. Iron is essential for efficient circulation and healthy blood, as are vitamin E (in wheatgerm, wholegrains, nuts, vegetable oils); folic acid (in yeast, liver, milk, green vegetables); vitamin B12 (in liver, meat, wholemeal flour, wheatgerm), and iodine (in seafoods, kelp, sea salt).

For steady nerves you need the following: vitamin B complex (yeast products, liver, wheatgerm); calcium (milk, cheese, parsley, yogurt); magnesium (salads, vegetables, greens, nuts, beans, lentils, wholegrains) and cobalt (sweetbreads, mushrooms, liver).

If you are a teenager or pregnant mum, you'll need extra calcium, vitamins A and D and iron. Smoking causes a lowering in the body's supply of C. A volatile nutrient at the best of times, vitamin C cannot be stored by the body, so an orange eaten last week will not help give you clear skin and resistance to disease today. Top up your 'C' supplies with citrus fruits (oranges, lemons, grapefruit), jacket potatoes, salads or drink a pure orange juice every day at breakfast.

If you're on the Pill, you could be suffering from vitamin B6 depletion. This vitamin is necessary for healthy skin and is involved in many bodily processes including protein metabolism. Good sources are liver, chicken, wholegrains, bananas. Liver also contains other B complex vitamins, so it's worth eating at least once a week. (Try it curried, braised with onions, or sliced and sautéed with sour cream.)

Calcium and magnesium work together as a natural tranquillizer. So, from a beauty standpoint they are vital in helping to control stress and insomnia, and beating stress-related symptoms like wrinkles, acne, allergies, and even obesity. Good sources? Milk and milk products for calcium (take calcium tablets if you can't stand them!); leafy vegetables, salads, lentils, wholegrains for magnesium.

# Diets for beauty

On these pages there are two diets: a 1000-calorie-a-day 'bikini' diet for an easy, fairly rapid weight loss, and a 1500-calorie-a-day diet for a slow but sure weight loss. Use the first diet for pre-holiday slimming, when you're in top form, the second for when you're feeling podgy and below par.

The 'bikini' diet is from *Leanline Cookery* by Hilda Woolf.

## 1000-calorie diet

Use skimmed milk in tea or coffee, no sugar. Drink water or low-calorie soft drinks, and the occasional glass of dry wine.

### DAY ONE

**Breakfast** Toast 2 slices slimmers' bread, spread with beef extract, top with a little grated Edam cheese and grill; tea or coffee.
**Lunch** Potato salad; 1 banana; tea or coffee.
**Supper** Smoked fish in spicy sauce; spinach; tea or coffee.

### DAY TWO

**Breakfast** 12gm (1 oz) bran cereal with small chopped grapefruit and sweetener; milk; slimmers' bread, toasted with beef extract. Tea or coffee.
**Lunch** Cheese salad; slimmers' apple snow; tea or coffee.
**Supper** Marinated grilled pork chop; spinach; fresh fruit salad; tea or coffee.

### DAY THREE

**Breakfast** As day one.
**Lunch** Spinach and tomato salad; 25gm (2 oz) hard cheese on 1 slice wholemeal toast; 1 pear; tea or coffee.
**Supper** Chicken marinated in piquant sauce; bean sprouts; stewed apple with orange juice; tea or coffee.

### DAY FOUR

**Breakfast** Juice of $\frac{1}{2}$ lemon diluted with water; 1 egg, poached on wholemeal bread; tea or coffee.
**Lunch** Potato salad; fresh fruit salad with yogurt; tea or coffee.
**Supper** 75gm (6 oz) lean chops or hamburger; 50gm (4 oz) courgettes, boiled; 25gm (2 oz) mushrooms, grilled; tomato, grilled; 1 banana with 12gm (1 oz) Edam cheese. Tea or coffee.

### DAY FIVE

**Breakfast** As day one.
**Lunch** As day one.
**Supper** Crispy vegetables in cheese and mustard sauce; Fresh fruit salad; tea or coffee.

### DAY SIX

**Breakfast** As day two.
**Lunch** Glass grapefruit or orange juice; 1 large egg, poached, on 1 slice slimmers' bread, toasted, with 12gm (1 oz) cheese, 1 tomato; tea or coffee.
**Supper** As day one.

### DAY SEVEN

**Breakfast** As day three.
**Lunch** As day two.
**Supper** Baked mackerel; broccoli; 1 apple; tea or coffee.

## 1500-calorie diet

You are allowed each day: 0.4 litre ($\frac{3}{4}$ pint) milk; 3 medium slices wholemeal bread; 5gm ($\frac{1}{2}$ oz) butter; raw sliced vegetables to nibble between meals; 1 glass dry wine each day.

### DAY ONE

**Breakfast** Baked egg nest; fruit juice; tea or coffee.
**Lunch** Salad with onion and yogurt dressing (2 spring onions, chopped and stirred into 1 carton of yogurt); beef extract drink.

**Supper** Celery and tomato starter; portion grilled white fish; 1 tablespoon mashed potato; 1 orange; wine, tea or coffee.

## DAY TWO

**Breakfast** Cottage eggs; wholewheat bread with honey; fruit juice; tea or coffee.
**Lunch** Spread 2 slices slimmers' bread with 1 teaspoon yogurt blended with grated cheese and horseradish sauce. Top with onion rings, tomato, cucumber. Green salad; tea or coffee.
**Supper** Slimmers' tomato soup; grilled liver (2 slices); 1 rasher grilled bacon; green vegetables; wine, tea or coffee.

## DAY TWO    (Alternative)

**Breakfast** Breakfast in a glass; slice of whole-wheat toast, butter and beef extract; tea or coffee.
**Lunch** As day one, plus 1 apple or orange.
**Supper** Half grapefruit; grilled chicken leg with carrots and cabbage; raspberry jelly; wine allowance, tea or coffee.

## DAY THREE

**Breakfast** Grapefruit juice; Devilled kidneys; slice of toast and butter; tea or coffee.
**Lunch** Glass of tomato juice; plus lunch served on day two.
**Supper** Clear soup; marinated grilled pork chop; 1 apple; wine allowance; tea or coffee.

## DAY FOUR

**Breakfast** As day one.
**Lunch** Large salad with dressing: 2 tablespoons natural yogurt with a pinch of curry powder; 25gm (2 oz) ham or other lean meat; apple; tea or coffee.
**Supper** Grilled sausage; mushroom omelette (2 eggs); green salad with lemon juice dressing; wine allowance, tea or coffee.

## DAY FIVE

**Breakfast** As day two.
**Lunch** Salad of grated onion, 1 tomato, 25gm (2 oz) shredded red cabbage and watercress topped with sliced egg, 25gm (2 oz) Edam cheese; tea or coffee.
**Supper** Clear vegetable soup; small portion grilled fish; 1 tablespoon mashed potato; mixed salad; orange sorbet; wine, tea or coffee.

## DAY SIX

**Breakfast** As day three.
**Lunch** As day one.
**Supper** 75gm (6 oz) casseroled stewing steak; boiled onion; carrots, french beans; unsweetened natural yogurt, wine allowance, tea or coffee.

## DAY SEVEN

**Breakfast** As day four.
**Lunch** As day two.
**Supper** As day one.

Underlined recipes on pp. 60-63

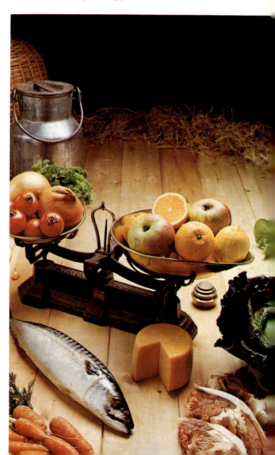

# Your body type

The art of being beautiful is in making the most of what you've got and learning to love your body. Luckily, it's now far less fashionable to be thin than it was five or six years ago: what counts is a healthy firm body, super posture and glowing skin. But this doesn't stop you aiming to improve your shape, as long as you stick within the confines of possibilities!

Your body type is determined by genetic influences and shaped by your environment, lifestyle and appetite. Below, you'll see the three main body shapes, but these are obviously fairly general, and your body is highly individual. The North European female type is the endomorph, and this is confirmed by surveys carried out by the large chain stores. We're often pear-shaped, with a fat tummy. But since the Pill became more generally used, many of us increased our bust measurement by 4 cm (2 inches).

Men aren't so easily categorized: they fall

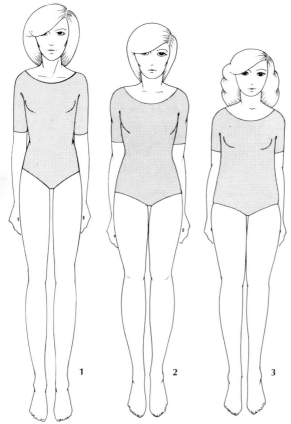

1       2       3

*1. The ectomorph. Lanky, slender and usually thin, these people have delicate bone structure, thin and stringy muscles. They rarely get fat (in fact have to watch that they don't become too thin) unless they overeat to extremes.*
*2. The mesomorph. These are the strong, muscular types with large bone and muscle development. They have big chests, small tums, well-developed muscles and big body joints. They sometimes become overweight. They are usually athletic.*
*3. The endomorph. They have a soft, round tum, usually bigger than the chest with small bones, hands and feet. They are most apt to become overweight.*

equally between the mesomorph and the endomorph categories, with a sprinkling of ectomorphs. But most men carry too much spare flesh.

To determine your own bone structure, strip to your undies and look at yourself in a long mirror. If your top half is noticeably smaller than your hips (look at the width between your hip-bones, not the flesh contours), and your hands and feet are small, then you come into the endomorph category. You should aim for a flat tummy (it *is* possible even though, according to psychologists, the endomorph is very food-and-comfort orientated), neat bustline, small waistline and trim hips. They'll never measure 86 cm (34 inches), but could be a neat 93 cm (36½ inches). You should not aim to be a skinny-hipped beauty. Depending on your height, you could weigh between 58 and 78 kilos (9 and 12 stone) for men, and 52 and 65 kilos (8 and 10 stone) for women.

If your shoulders are broad, your bosom full and your midriff flat (or potentially flat under the extra weight), then you are a mesomorph. Your bones are sturdy, your hips broad. You should aim to be well covered but firm all over and perhaps link this idea to exercise, since the mesomorphs are usually sports-orientated. You should not aim to be thin or weigh 52 kilos (8 stone). Depending on your height, you should weigh between 65 and 87 kilos (10 and 13½ stone) for men and 58 and 71 kilos (9 and 11 stone) for women.

If you are tall, with delicate bone structure and remember being called 'lanky' when you were a teenager, then you are the ectomorph type. Measure your wrist if your body is too fat to judge bone structure accurately: it will be around 15 cm (6 inches) for women or 23 cm (9 inches) for men. If you're a fat ectomorph, then you're probably very greedy since this type doesn't often become overweight. You should aim to be slim and lithe. Around 65-75 kilos (10-11½

stone) for men or 52-60 kilos (8-9½ stone) for women. You should not aim to be a voluptuous Boticelli beauty since the extra fat will just look ugly on your delicate frame.

Once you've established just what is practical for you, then your best guide towards achieving this is your mirror. Check your shape as often as you can: perhaps two or three times a week. Concentrate on the good points about your body. If you are following a diet or exercise programme to achieve the best possible potential for your own particular shape, then note encouraging signs: flatter tum, improved posture, slimmer legs. Don't dwell on the things that will never be altered, like your hip bones, your small bustline or your full ribcage.

The most beautiful women in the world are never model-girl perfect, but they do know how to become *bien dans la peau*, the French way of saying 'happy in your skin'.

## Checking your weight

There are lots of weight-height ratio charts available for a simple check on your desirable weight. The trouble is that most of these are very generous, based on data used by life-insurance companies to check potential clients. Most of us cheat when we read them! If you consult a chart, be realistic about your body frame.

A healthy weight for you will depend on the life you lead as well as your body type. Don't be skinny if your life is centred around entertaining and you adore good food. You'll make yourself, and others, miserable. If in doubt, check with your doctor, especially if you intend going on a diet such as the ones on pp. 10 and 11.

## The psychology of shape

Recently, several books have been published on body type and the psychological make-up of individuals. Check yourself for

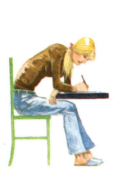
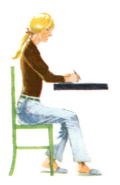
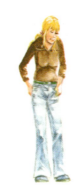
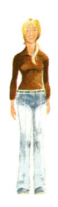

▲ If you sit badly (left) your spine is curved which will lead to backache, and possibly even disc trouble. Your tummy is compressed, concertina-fashion, producing a bulging midriff! Correct posture (right) seat is well back, spine straight, legs at 90° angle.

▲ If you stand badly, (left) your shoulders are slouched straining the back and neck. Legs are wobbly, tummy sticking out. Correct posture (right): tummy is tucked in, legs straight, back relaxed but straight, and shoulders down. Head is held high to discourage double chin forming, arms are relaxed.

these characteristics (but don't take the findings too seriously!). If you have a thin body, with sunken chest and head thrown forward, you need friends, lots of social activity, hate being alone. You're impulsive. With a short, thick body, hunched shoulders and forward-curving spine you're a martyr, and feel you're under pressure. You're stubborn too, and often suppress anger. A straight, rigid body with stiff shoulders may mean you're pushy, serious, determined, but long for love and support. You find it very hard to relax!

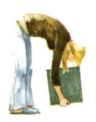
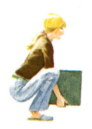

▲ No wonder so many people have back trouble: most of us use the spine to take the strain of lifting. On the left, the spine is curved, no use is made of the legs. Correct posture (right): the thigh muscles were built to take the strain of lifting, your back wasn't.

## How your lifestyle shapes your body

Before tackling an exercise programme to improve your shape, look at the way your lifestyle shapes your body. Every single time you use a desk that's too low, an ironing board that's too high or sit hunched in an easy chair watching television, you are coaxing limbs, muscles, tissue into unnatural shapes: possibly permanently.

Look around: you can usually spot a man or woman who works hunched over a low desk all day: their shoulders are rounded, head poked forward. Dentists are often occupationally deformed workers: bending all day, mostly to one side with the weight of the body pressed heavily on one leg, most dentists eventually become stooped. Here's a guide to the working conditions that will do most for your figure.

1. Tables and desks should be at a comfortable height: sitting on a chair, with back straight, feet flat on the floor, your bent elbows should just touch the table-top.

2. Working surfaces in kitchens and workshops should be at wrist-height when you stand close to them, with one foot forward, shoulders relaxed. As you work, your shoulders will remain low and back, and not hunched (sciatica, headaches and migraine are all associated with hunched shoulders!). The counter-level in a store should be the same height, and you can adjust your own level if the counter is too high by using a footstool. Why not, otherwise you may be working at the same bad level for six hours a day!

3. Equipment such as paperwork, files, kitchen tools, bench tools should be within easy reach if you are using it as you work. A swivel chair can prevent painful body twisting, slanting shoulders, backache.

4. Shoes should be comfortable and the heel-height and sole-height be balanced so that you don't have to lean backwards to prevent yourself falling over. This is a vital point for pregnant mums.

5. Beds should be firm and large enough to allow easy movement. A firm bed allows you to relax muscles evenly, otherwise a hip, shoulder or leg may sink into the mattress making other muscles work hard all night to support the body-level.

6. Mirrors on dressing tables should be at a comfortable height. Use them, too, to check your posture. Shop windows are also useful for this.

7. Cars are perhaps the worst body-twisters of all. Most are very badly designed with little or no support for the lower back. A small cushion can help counteract this, and make sure you adjust the seat so your knees are bent comfortably, hands and arms relaxed with shoulders down and back as you drive. Make sure your vision is good over the wheel to prevent cricks in the neck.

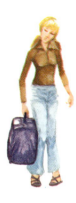

*Many women spend a lot of time slumped over their shopping bags (left). The body is out of balance with one shoulder dipping at an alarming angle. Ideally the body should be balanced (below). Either make an effort to keep your back straight, your posture erect, or divide your shopping equally between your two hands.*

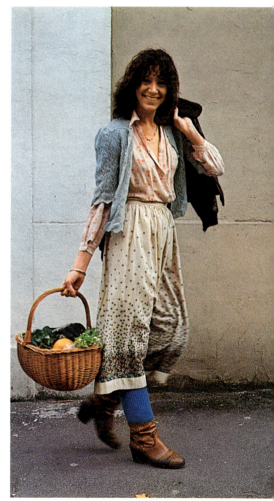

# Massage and sauna

Regular massage helps keep your skin supple, muscles toned and body relaxed. Massage won't make you lose weight, but it will encourage the dispersal of stubborn fat tissue in problem spots like thighs, upper arms and tummy. Most important, massage helps 'iron out' the aches, creaks and stiffness of everyday living: . posture, shoulder and back pain, sore limbs, stress are all helped by regular massage. But such luxurious beauty care needn't be expensive. You can indulge in a weekly massage at home—with the help of a friend. Or, you can give *yourself* a daily massage using a good body lotion or cream. After bathing is the best time when your skin is slightly warm and you feel relaxed. Here's a step-by-step massage treatment.

1. Spread oil over subject's back, place hands on his shoulders. Gently press thumbs above shoulder blades, palms lightly onto shoulders and make circular movements. Repeat 20 times. Now stroke hands from shoulders to spine. Repeat 20 times.

*You need:* body massage cream or oil (see recipes opposite); soft towel; paper tissues to absorb oil residue; a warm room (bathroom or bedroom).

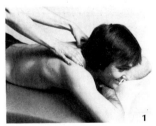

2. Place hands in position as shown. Now make strong strokes across his back, working down towards the waist. Repeat 20 times.

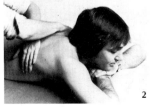

3. Place hands either side of your friend's right leg. Now make firm strokes downward to the ankle. Repeat 10 times with each leg. Now make similar strokes to those used in 2. across back of leg from thigh to ankle.

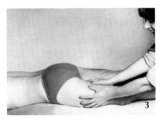

4. Cup hands and place them across his calf. Move hands alternately across calf in a steady movement, working down towards ankle level. Repeat 30 times. Now work extra oil between toes, balls and arches of feet.

5. Clasp his arm as shown and lift to a vertical position. Now gently massage from wrist to armpit all around the arm. Lower arm for a few seconds, pick up hand and massage more oil between fingers, working from fingertips to wrist. Repeat with other arm and hand.

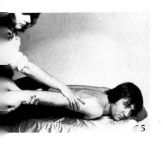

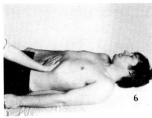

2. across body from midriff to tummy. Repeat 30 times.

6

5. Spread oil on partner's tummy and massage in circular movements all around navel with the palm of your hand. With both hands repeat the strokes used in

7. End the massage with more soothing shoulder and throat strokes, placing fingertips at

throat as shown and working outwards in circular movements. Repeat 20 times. Blot surplus oil with tissues and allow your friend to rest quietly for 15 minutes before dressing.

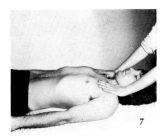

7

## Oils and lotions

Baby oil, with a few drops of perfume essence added, makes a good inexpensive massage oil. Or you can use baby lotion for a creamier, less messy effect. Some beauticians and aromatherapists, who specialize in massage using essential oils and particular pressure points, will even send body oils by post. Don't forget: be lavish with the lotion you use as it will quickly be absorbed by the warm skin. For men, baby oil plus a few drops of their favourite aftershave or toilet water makes a good fresh-smelling lotion.

## After your massage

You'll feel relaxed, a bit sleepy. If you can, try to rest quietly for at least 15 minutes. If you have your massage at night, you can curl up in a warm bed and sleep peacefully. Next morning, you'll feel great and your skin will be as soft as silk.

## Remember

Massage is particularly useful during the weeks before a holiday in the sun. It helps prepare the skin and makes it more supple and able to cope with drying salt water and hot sun. If you are pregnant, massage your skin all over very lightly from the very first moment you hear the good news to help prevent stretch marks.

## Sauna

Sauna baths are relaxing, refreshing and will certainly help cleanse your skin. The dry heat of the Swedish and Finnish-style wooden sauna cabins you find at health clubs and health farms is less drastic for both your own comfort and your skin than the wet, clammy heat of a turkish bath or cabinet. Ideally, you should stay in the cabinet for short periods (two to five minutes), with a cool shower between each session to wash away the perspiration and grime forced to the surface of your pores by the temperature.

The best times for a sauna are in the spring, when your skin is grimy after a winter of thick clothes, central heating and city life, and in the autumn, when the remnants of your summer tan are beginning to look 'yellow' and your skin needs freshening-up.

The worst times for a sauna are when you're below par, have been following a crash diet or have just had your hair re-styled! Seriously, you should never stay too long in the sauna cabinet or go in at all if you have a history of high blood pressure, heart trouble, respiratory diseases or very dry skin.

# Fresh is beautiful

Beauty should always start with the basics: being fresh and clean is important for your own morale as well as your looks and your relationships with other people. But freshness should not be an antiseptic state and a clean body should smell like a body, not a hospital operating theatre. What's more, certain products such as vaginal deodorants have been shown to be unnecessary, and possibly even dangerous. Certain types of micro-organism living on the surface of the skin do a very useful protective job, and they should be allowed to function.

The sweat glands cover the body concentrated at around 650 glands every 2 sq cm (1 sq inch) from your scalp to the soles of your feet. There are two types: the eccrine glands which are present over almost all the body and secrete a clear, thin, watery fluid (about 99 per cent water, 1 per cent inorganic salts.) This fluid is odourless as it emerges, but it picks up odour on contact with the air. The apocrine glands are situated in the anal and pubic areas, underarms, tummy, breasts. They secrete a thicker, odourless liquid which is attacked by bacteria and rapidly becomes rancid-smelling. It's more pronounced if the sweat is stimulated by nerves, anxiety or desire than if it's simply triggered off by hot weather.

An all-over wash with a bland soap, which should be rinsed off very thoroughly, once or twice a day in hot weather will cope adequately with most perspiration. Use a deodorant or antiperspirant under your arms (the roll-on kind are longer-lasting and more effective than aerosols) or, if you are allergic to the aluminium salts they contain, try a solution of cider vinegar in water: 1 tablespoon to $\frac{1}{2}$ litre (1 pint) water. The same brew is smashing for hot, sweaty feet too.

If you have to work in a hot, crowded office keep a deodorant at work and always wear cotton undies, shirts and natural-fibre sweaters or dresses. Men should avoid nylon underwear, particularly pants, which cause a sticky build-up of perspiration and can even lead to spots. Wash clothes regularly, change socks and tights every day and go barefoot in hot weather if you possibly can. Stockings are more hygienic for women than tights.

During a period, be even more careful about daily washing. Change cotton pants several times a day. You should not need to use an 'intimate' deodorant. Shaving body hair is a personal thing, but there is no doubt that underarm hair does increase body odour, so if you prefer to let yours grow naturally, then wash the area more often.

Diet is an important factor in controlling B.O. Green vegetables, particularly parsley, contain chlorophyll, which is a natural deodorant. 'Smelly' foods include highly spiced curries, garlic, cheese and milk-based foods. If you've had a highly spiced meal at night, drink plenty of water to 'dilute' the smell and concentrate on salad foods the next day.

## Recipes for freshness

1. Breath freshener: grind a few caraway seeds and mix with 1 tablespoon crushed cloves, 1 tablespoon ground cinnamon, and 1 tablespoon crushed nutmeg. Mix into a large glass of sherry. Use the brew diluted in water as it's very strong.
2. Deodorant: mix a few drops each of lavender oil, patchouli oil and oil of camphor. Add to 0.25 litres ($\frac{1}{2}$ pint) water.

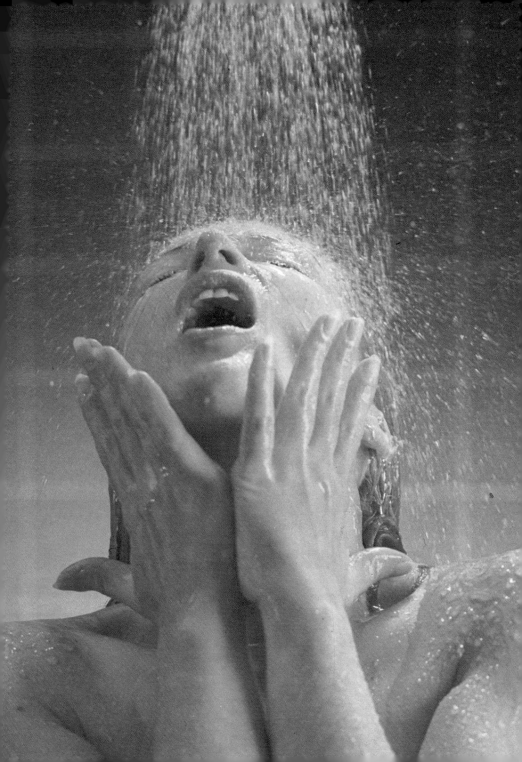

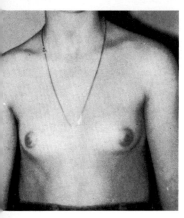

1. For the very flat-chested a breast augmentation operation can often be highly successful.

2. The first stage of the operation is to make an incision beneath the natural contour of the breast.

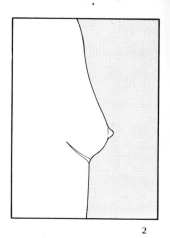

1

2

# Cosmetic surgery

Nowadays, there is a great deal of interest in cosmetic surgery to correct really severe beauty problems. For some people it can be a real psychological boon, transforming their personality as well as appearance. But it should not be undertaken without the fullest possible consideration and consultation with an expert in the field.

The first step is to consult your family doctor. If he or she is unsympathetic, then your local hospital will be able to put you in touch with a consultant. Beware of surgeons who advertise their clinics in magazines. Insist on having your problem investigated thoroughly, and get everything explained to you in detail before you get as far as the operation itself. A good surgeon will dissuade you from having the operation if he thinks it's unnecessary.

Here's a guide to the most popular cosmetic surgery and what it entails.
1. Full face lift (rhytiodoplasty): The skin is smoothed out and tightened, with the surplus eased out towards small scars in front and behind ears. Bandages are re-moved 24-48 hours after the operation and the patient usually leaves the clinic within three days. Stitches are removed on the ninth or tenth day. Bruising and reddening of the skin lasts for two to three weeks. The results last for about 10-15 years, when the sags start again. Around 65 years is the maximum age for this operation and three lifts are the limit.
2. Dermabrasion: the top layer of skin is removed from the face in this operation to help clear the scars of severe acne. When the bandages are removed a day or two later the skin starts to form a yellow healing 'crust'. Gradually, new skin is formed and in about two months the face returns to normal.
3. Nose remodelling (rhinoplasty): this operation involves a lot of discomfort and takes about three or four months to recover from. The patient is under local anaesthetic and incisions are made high up inside the nostrils so no scars are visible. Bone and cartilege can be removed or flattened, and fleshy areas remodelled.

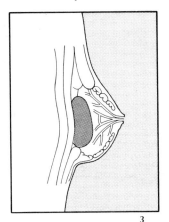

3. The mammary gland and breast tissue are lifted and a silicone jelly-filled bag is placed behind the breast gland against the chest wall.

4. The incision is sutured and the scar is covered by the breast's natural shape.

5. The girl's fuller breasts improve her figure, but the operation has not lessened their sensitivity or removed the possibility of breast-feeding.

3

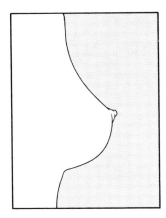

4

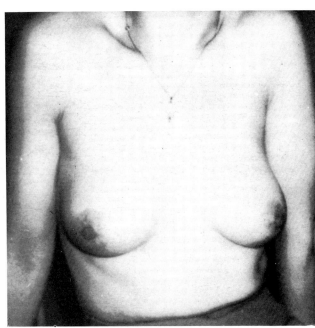

5

4. Eyelid surgery (blepharoplasty): this kind of surgery helps smooth out wrinkles in the upper eyelids, crows' feet, bulges in the lower eyelids and bags. Eye-bag operations are usually very successful and don't need re-doing at all. No scars are visible. The patient stays in the clinic for around two to three days, stitches are removed, and the bruising heals after about three weeks.

5. Breast surgery (mammoplasty): there are two kinds of breast operation: reduction and augmentation. The former is a radical operation with nipple-resetting and scarring which fades gradually. The latter is less difficult and involves a small incision under the breasts and the implanting of a bag-like pad containing soft silicone jelly. The bag is placed between the chest wall and the under surface of the breast gland, so the sensitivity and natural look of the breast is not impaired and breast feeding is still possible. For breast reduction, patients should be under 50 and in good health. The length of stay in the clinic is about five days for reducing, three days for enlarging. Scarring starts to heal after about two weeks, but patients for both operations must take things easily for about six weeks.

6. Tummy, buttock and thigh lifts. These operations are more serious.

# Exercise for beauty

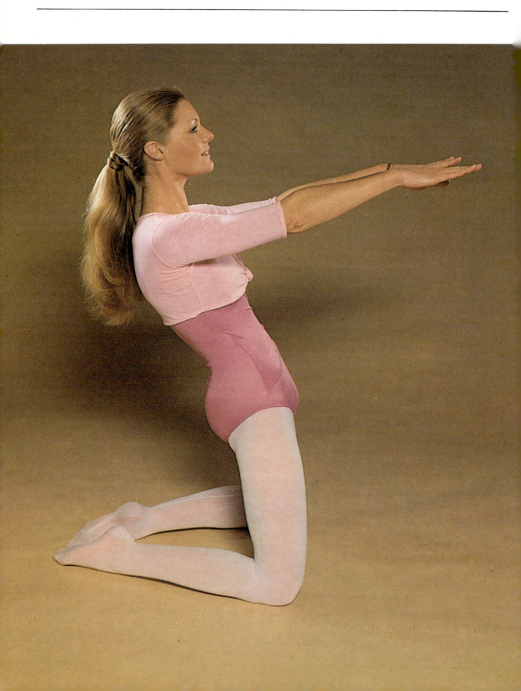

The benefits of regular, controlled exercise are tremendous, ranging from an improved shape to a much more relaxed outlook on life. But it's often difficult to find an exercise programme that is easy and pleasant to follow, doesn't become boring and doesn't involve a lot of time. For no exercise routine will do a scrap of good unless it's followed regularly. Frantic physical jerks once a month are tiring, but not beautifying!

Jo Kemp, an ex-ballet dancer who runs a successful London exercise studio, has devised an exercise routine that's fun to follow, helps streamline the body and relax the mind. It's based on yoga asanas, with carefully controlled, slowly executed movements which are not tiring, boring or

◀ *Thigh stretcher. Kneel on the floor with knees slightly apart, feet touching, arms straight out in front with palms down. Inhale. Tuck bottom and tummy in. Lean back slowly keeping trunk straight as you exhale. Hold position. Inhale, then come back to starting position. Repeat 3-10 times.*

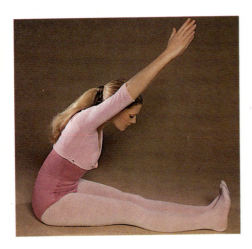

▲ *Tummy toner. Sit on the floor, feet together, with toes pointing at the ceiling. Raise arms above head, palms pressed together. Inhale. Tuck in your tum and lean forward slowly, exhaling on the way down. Touch toes— or ankles! Repeat 5 times, hold toes (or ankles) and try to stretch a little further.*

dangerous for novices. What's more, Jo's routine, which includes correct breathing techniques, leaves you feeling envigorated instead of exhausted. The exercises make you aware of your body-tone, muscles and posture, so you start to move much more gracefully, eat more sensibly and enjoy life more.

Elimination processes are helped too, so your body feels less podgy and much sleeker, even if you don't need to lose much weight. After doing the exercises regularly for a few days, most of Jo's students find that they can throw away laxative pills and sleeping tablets!

Obviously, it's better if you can go along to a studio like Jo's to get expert instruction, but if time is precious, you can follow Jo's exercise routine at home.

Set aside 10-15 minutes each day for your exercise session, preferably when you are alone. Jo advises tackling the movements when your body is relaxed after a warm, but not hot, bath. It's vital to be comfortable, so wear a leotard and tights or a T-shirt and pair of pants or stretchy shorts. Jeans are not suitable since they restrict your movements and prevent you from controlling your breathing properly.

## Breathing technique

Before you start, practise the breathing technique. Stand straight, feet slightly apart, toes turned inwards. Now place both hands, fingers spread, on your tummy. Breathe in, deeply, through your mouth, feeling your tummy expand as you do so. Now breathe out blowing the air through your lips, making a whistling noise, and feeling your tummy flatten; until all the air has been squeezed out of your lungs and your tummy is almost concave. This breathing method is used in all the exercises, and will feel strange at first, so practise as often as possible. It's a super tummy-toning exercise in itself!

▼ *Head rolls for neck tension.* Sit cross-legged, hands on your knees. Inhale; now exhale as you lean your head to one side, then back, then to the other side in circular movements. Keep your body straight, tummy tucked in. Inhale on completing one 'circle', then exhale. Repeat 10 times.

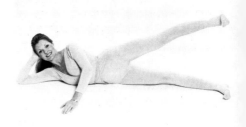

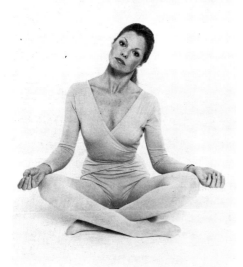

▲ *Leg raises for thighs and legs.* Lie on your side, one arm supporting your head, the other hand flat on the floor in front of you. Inhale. Now exhale and raise your leg slowly making sure that toes point forwards. Pause; inhale; then exhale as you lower your leg. Repeat 10 times with each leg.

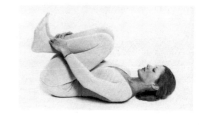

▼ *Shoulder stretch for shoulders and arms.* Lie on your back on the floor, feet apart, knees relaxed. Inhale and drop your chin to your chest. Now exhale and hold your tummy in as you try to reach for the ceiling with your right hand. Feel your tummy to make sure it's flat. Repeat with the other hand. Repeat 20 times.

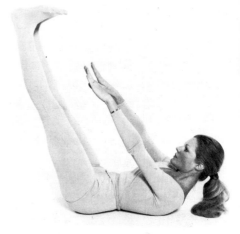

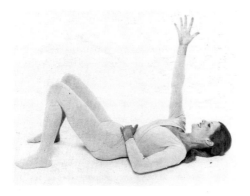

▲ *Tummy tightener for midriff, tummy and thighs.* Lie on your back. Inhale. Exhale and slowly raise your knees onto your chest, clasping your ankles. Inhale. Exhale and stretch your legs upwards, and your hands towards them with arms straight, lifting your head slightly as you do so. Inhale. Exhale and lower your legs and arms slowly. Inhale. Repeat 5-10 times.

▼ *Pelvis tightener. Lie on your back, knees raised and feet apart with knees relaxed and hands palms-uppermost at your sides. Inhale. Exhale as you tighten your bottom and raise your pelvis off the floor. Inhale. Exhale, and lower your pelvis, squeezing all the air out of your tum. Repeat 15 times.*

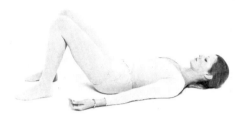

▼ *Bottom trimmer. Kneel on the floor, hands and legs slightly apart and inhale as you bring your right knee up to touch your nose, lowering your head to meet it. Now exhale. Inhale and stretch your leg upwards and back and look up to the ceiling. Exhale. Inhale and bring your knee back to touch your nose. Exhale. Inhale and lower your knee to the floor. Repeat 5 times with each leg.*

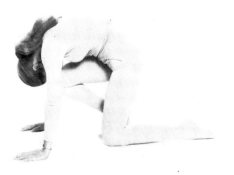

▶ *Posture pose. Stand with back straight, feet slightly apart, palms pressed together, elbows out. Now inhale, pushing your tummy out. Exhale, squeezing all the air out of your tummy, pressing your palms together, tucking in your bottom and relaxing your shoulders at the same time. Inhale and relax. Repeat 15 times.*

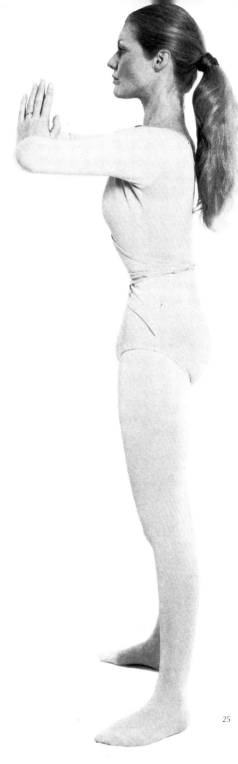

# Be a sport

The most enjoyable way to keep in trim is to find time in your schedule, however busy you are, for sport. Whatever your age-group, sex or occupation, there is a sport that's right for you. As well as helping to tone your muscles and trim your body, sport is a valuable way of relieving tension and stress. But doctors warn that it's important to take it easy at first, especially if you decide to tackle a physically demanding sport after a long period of inactivity. It's unwise, for instance, to play a tough game of squash after a lazy holiday or a spell in hospital: break yourself in gently with some long walks, jogging and a sensible, healthy diet. Jogging itself should be approached cautiously: try combining 100 jogging steps with 100 walking steps and gradually increasing your distance and speed. Women should make sure they wear a good supporting bra when jogging, as breast tissue can be stretched by the bouncing movement.

## Swimming

Don't let swimming become your summer exercise only: find a local pool and go swimming once or twice a week to develop a whole range of beauty assets from trim tummy muscles to a super bustline. Swimming helps exercise the pectoral muscles which support the bustline, does great things for legs, arms, breathing and posture. It's also cheap and can be fitted into a lunch hour, evening or weekend very easily indeed. Everyone should learn how to swim. If you can't, then combine lessons with a valuable, low-priced beauty treatment.

Recommended for everyone, particularly those who can't undertake more strenuous exercise.

## Judo and martial arts

Judo teaches balance, control, grace, posture, breathing and tones thigh, arm and tummy muscles. It's ideal if you're in an office or shop job where you may be unnaturally hunched for many hours in the day. You don't need to be a toughie to be successful at judo: the holds and falls demand technique rather than strength. Most towns have judo and karate clubs. Another Eastern technique catching on rapidly in Europe is tai chi, which involves slow ballet-like series of movements. It's graceful and fun.

Recommended for children and teenagers who want to develop good muscle control and older people in sedentary or stationary jobs.

## Squash

Although it's sometimes difficult to find a vacancy at a squash club since the game has become so popular, it's worthwhile persevering. For squash exercises all the major muscle groups in a very short time. A session of 40 minutes provides as much exercise as a round of golf or 3-4 hours jogging. It's excellent for legs, arms, posture, breathing control, and general stamina and fitness. If you have a job, you can fit squash into a lunch hour easily: if you lead a busy life at home, an early morning game will leave the rest of the day free. It needs regular practise though and should never be played after a heavy meal.

Recommended for housewives and business-people.

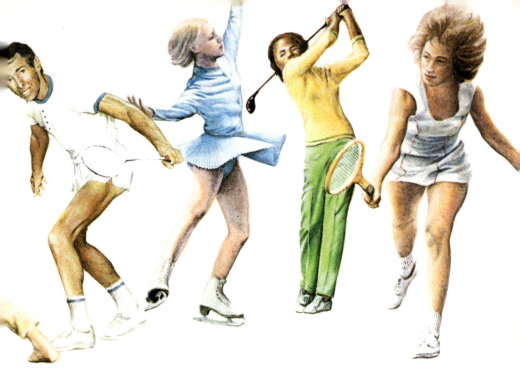

### Skating

Skating teaches grace, poise, good posture and body control. It helps tone leg, ankle, thigh and tummy muscles and midriff. It is also exhilarating and the cold atmosphere of the rink helps blow away the cobwebs of work and home life. To learn properly, it's wise to have lessons at a local rink. You do not have to be a tiny tot to learn to skate. Skating rinks normally have good social facilities for adult members and it costs about the same amount as going to the cinema, though it's much more fun.

Recommended for office and factory workers; anyone in a job that's tough on the feet, since skating helps strengthen feet and ankles.

### Golf

Choose golf as your sport if you want a trim waistline and trunk, strong arms and wrists and good general body tone. It's a sport for loners who enjoy pitting their wits against the ball and have one or two afternoons or mornings free each week. Women are coming more into the sport since the tight rules and regulations of many male-dominated clubs are being relaxed. The main danger? Too many drinks after the game. You can replace the calories used during a game of golf with just 6 short drinks and a sandwich afterwards.

Recommended for older people with enough time and funds to enjoy this sometimes expensive sport; anyone who works in a stuffy atmosphere.

### Tennis

Tennis isn't just a glamorous sport, it's also very effective for exercising legs, arms, waistline, and tummy. The big tennis tournaments usually inspire thousands of amateurs to take it up, but then their enthusiasm fades. However, indoor courts exist for winter games, so tennis can be an all-the-year-round sport. Join a club for the best social and playing conditions. Aim to play at least once or twice a week. Invest in a good lightweight racket, good tennis shoes, and use them!

Recommended for all sedentary types, especially women. Note: watching a tennis match on TV burns off 1.4 calories a minute, playing in one burns 9 calories a minute!

# Exercises while you work

The most efficient and beneficial kind of exercise is the regular kind. So, what better than to combine easy exercises with other things, like work, for instance? Many physiotherapists are convinced that gentle exercise is better for you than physical jerks, and certainly, if you are unaccustomed to regular exercise, sports and daily keep-fit sessions can be a disaster. That's why doctors and fitness experts who treat hospital patients use isometric exercises. These exercises have two great benefits: they can be performed sitting down, in that office chair, for instance, and they are gentle.

How do they work? The word 'iso' means 'equal' and 'metric' means 'measurement'. In isometric exercises, muscles are toned and exercised by an equal, measured contraction against an immoveable object, such as the floor, a pile of books or a wastepaper basket. This contraction (usually to a slow count of six) strengthens the muscle without taxing heart, lungs, or respiratory system; in other words you don't get puffed. When the muscle is toned, then the surrounding flesh becomes firm and lithe.

How can they fit into your beauty programme? Easily! Very little effort is required for isometrics. What's more, they can provide an additional, frequent way of toning problem areas. For instance, if you know that a big bottom is your main figure problem, yet you have to sit at a typewriter all day, then 20 six-second isometric contractions on your buttock muscles every hour will certainly help streamline your seat.

Here are eight isometric exercises, for eight common problem areas. Pick out the ones that apply to you, and repeat them as often as possible throughout the day. In less than a week, you will see a noticeable improvement, especially if you combine them with the exercises on p. 22.

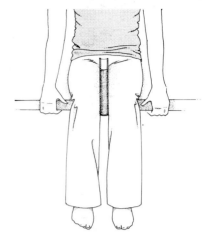

For bottom and inside thighs sit on a hard chair—remove that cushion—feet on the floor, back straight, knees apart. Now place a book between your knees and press them together hard, as if you were trying to crush the book. Count to six slowly while you hold the contraction. Then relax.

For legs sit with your back straight, clasping a metal wastepaper basket between your calves. Squeeze your legs together hard, count six slowly, then relax. Now place your feet inside the basket and push outwards hard, count six. Now relax.

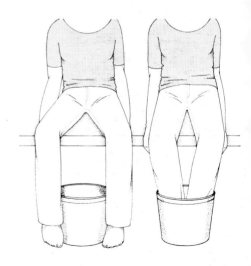

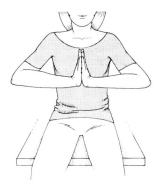

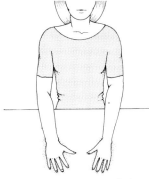

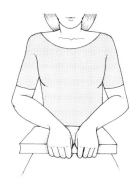

or pectoral muscles—the muscles above the breast that hold and lift your bosom—sit or stand with your back straight, place palms together in front of your chest, elbows up. Now push hard for a slow count of six and relax.

For upper arms sit at a desk or table, back straight, feet together, place the palms of your hands on the desk-top, about 4 cm (2 inches) apart. Now press down as hard as you can. Hold the contraction for a count of six. Relax. Now place palms flat underneath the table, and repeat the exercise.

For wrists and forearms sit comfortably and hold a thick, strong book at arms' length in both hands, positioning your hands as if you were attempting to tear it in half. Now pull one hand towards you, the other away from you at the same time. Hold the contraction for a count of six, then relax.

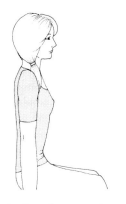

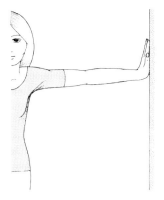

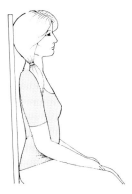

For back and tummy sit comfortably on a wooden chair, feet slightly apart, back straight. Now grip the seat of the chair with your hands. With arms straight pull in your tummy and pull against the chair seat hard. Hold for a count of six, then relax. Excellent for flabby, tense executives.

For arms, shoulders and back sit near a convenient wall and place the palm of one hand flat against it, keeping your arm perfectly straight and at right-angles to the wall. Now push hard, counting six slowly. Relax, and repeat with the other arm and hand.

For double chin and neck muscles sit in a high-backed chair, with your seat well back, hands on the arms of the chair or in your lap and feet firmly on the floor. Now press your back against the chair and push. Hold for a count of six, relax.

# All about your hair

Hair grows at the rate of about 1 cm ($\frac{1}{2}$ inch) a month from the follicle, which is situated in the epidermis. Although hair itself is a dead substance, the root is kept very much alive. The hairshaft is constructed from keratin, a form of protein, which is synthesized by the body from the protein foods we eat. Between the follicle and the shaft are the sebaceous glands. These secrete the sebum which runs down the hairshaft to give suppleness and gloss. If these glands become over-active for any reason, such as hormonal activity during puberty, then the hair will become greasier. If they are blocked by dirt or dandruff flakes or the glands become less active, then the hair will become dryer. Long hair is often dry at the ends because the sebum cannot run far enough down the hairshaft to keep the hair glossy.

## Pigmentation

The natural colour of your hair is inherited from your family and is formed by the inter-action of amino acids with melanin, a pigment that's also present in the skin. Dark hair is rich in cobalt, copper and iron, red hair in molybdenum, blonde hair in titanium, and white hair in nickel. Naturally, we need

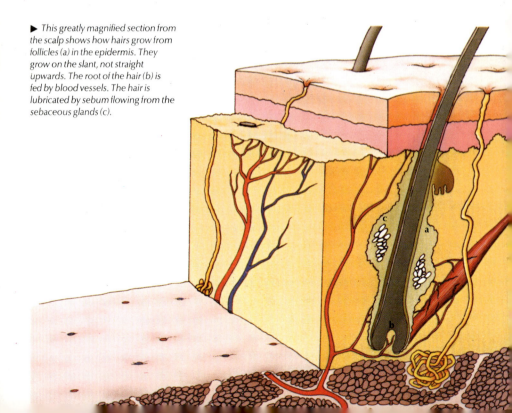

▶ This greatly magnified section from the scalp shows how hairs grow from follicles (a) in the epidermis. They grow on the slant, not straight upwards. The root of the hair (b) is fed by blood vessels. The hair is lubricated by sebum flowing from the sebaceous glands (c).

# How to cut your own hair

If you have a simple style like this popular bob cut, you can keep it in trim yourself. The best type of hair for home-trimming is the straight, fairly thick type with natural body. Don't attempt it if your hair is very fine or curly.

You will need two mirrors to give yourself a good back view, opaque tape, sharp hair-trimming scissors, clips and a tail-comb.

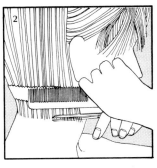

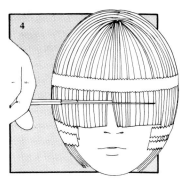

of short cuts and don't take up too much hair or you may get an uneven result.

3. Comb down the side and fringe hair from the central parting and fix it in place with a series of strips of tape, one each

5. Remove tape, check line of fringe and replace tape for extra trimming if necessary. Check for straggly ends and whisps of hair all over, particularly at nape of neck. Remove tape, damp hair again.

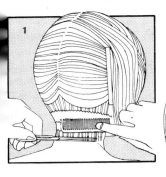

1. Wash and condition your hair as shown on p. 33. Comb out the hair and make a centre parting from the forehead to the nape of the neck. Comb away the side hair and clip it back out of the way. Now comb down the back hair from a horizontal parting about 4 cm (2 inches) above the nape of the neck. Place a strip of tape above the cutting line and trim the hair away evenly. Comb down another layer of hair and repeat. Keep going until the back hair is nicely lined up.

2. Comb hair down from the clips on the right side of your hair, tape in place and cut to match the back hair. Use a series

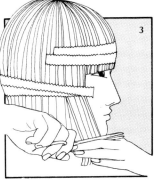

to secure the fringe, the crown and the side hair to ear level. Keep checking in the mirror that your head is level as you work and cut the hair to slope slightly downwards, so that it is longer and reaches to chin level in the front. Repeat with the other side, matching lengths carefully by bringing front side hair forwards.

4. Comb fringe forward, secure with tape and cut, allowing for 'shrinkage' as hair dries.

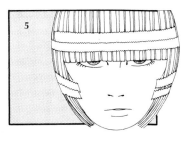

6. Blow-dry hair following instructions on p. 36, lifting from the root and curling fringe and sides under.

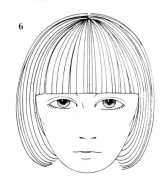

to take in these minerals in the food we eat to keep hair colour true. If you turn white or grey overnight blame your enzymes: a sudden shock can cause a blockage in the very complicated enzyme process that controls pigmentation.

## Caring for your hair

Shampoo your hair the day before it starts to look tacky. The frequent washing doesn't encourage greasiness although really rough scalp-rubbing will stimulate the sebaceous glands, so you should be gentle. This applies to your shampoo choice too: pick the mildest shampoo you can find as harsh detergent will strip natural conditioning oils from your hair.

Conditioners are useful for hard-to-handle hair and essential if you blow-dry your style into shape. But don't apply too much, and do rinse thoroughly, as some conditioners cause build-up on the hairshaft and attract dirt particles.

On holiday you should rinse your hair thoroughly with cold water after swimming and allow it to dry naturally (but not in hot sunshine). Salt and sand particles will lodge under the overlapping 'tiles' and eventually make the hairshaft snap if they are not removed.

Other hair horrors are heated rollers, tongs, metal rollers with bristles, central heating and woolly hats! Use heated rollers covered with tissue sparingly: never more than three times a week. A perm is less damaging than twice-daily curl-ups with rollers or tongs. Choose plain cheap plastic rollers if you roller-set your hair and hold them in place with a smooth-ended hairpin or plastic pin. Never roll them too tightly, and don't let your hairdresser do so either,

▼ *When the hair is in top condition the 'tiles' lie smoothly in place giving a glossy, healthy look.*

▼ *Too much brushing, heat or salt water can damage the overlapping keratin 'tiles' on the hairshaft.*

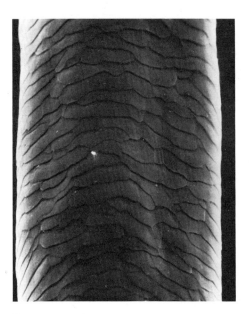

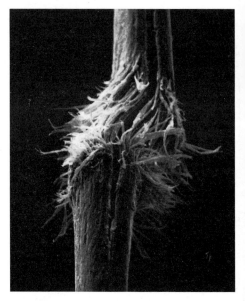

## Step-by-step shampoo guide

1. Using a spray attachment on the taps, wet hair thoroughly with hand-hot water.

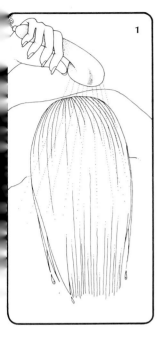

2. Pour a little shampoo into your hand—not onto your hair.

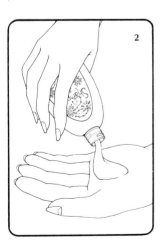

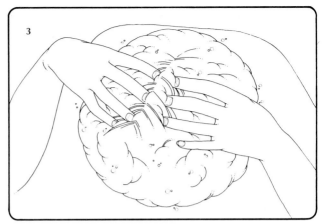

3. Starting at the roots, rub in gently with fingertips and let shampoo run down to the ends of the hair.

4. Rinse thoroughly until hair 'squeaks' and wrap in a towel to soak up moisture.

5. Apply conditioner or rinse hair in cool water with 1 teaspoon lemon juice (blonde hair) or vinegar (dark hair). Comb out with wide-gauge comb.

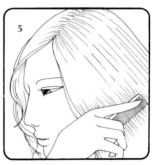

6. Rinse thoroughly, spraying from crown to ends. Towel-dry and wash comb in disinfectant.

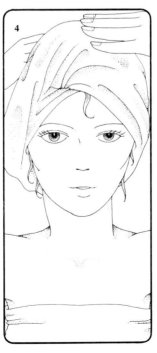

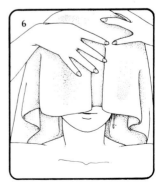

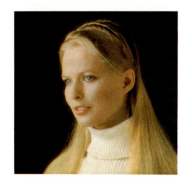

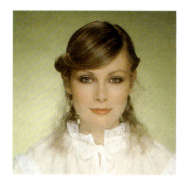

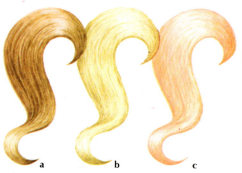

a          b          c

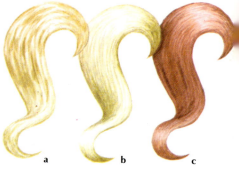

a          b          c

▲ *If your hair is naturally blonde, fine and lank, add body and thickness with a colourant. Honey blonde (a) would add golden lights to your natural shade. Try light blonde highlights (b) to give your hair a Scandinavian blonde look with minimal regrowth problems. Red highlights (c) can only be added in the salon, but are very attractive.*

▲ *Don't despair if your hair is naturally mousey, as this is the simplest colour to tint successfully. Blonde highlights (a) can be put in at home to add light, body, sex-appeal. Or you could have your hair lightened one or two shades then toned to ash-blonde (b). Pre-lightened hair can also be toned to a reddish-blonde shade (c).*

since hair stretches when wet, shrinks when dry. If you work in a centrally-heated office the combination of the warmth and dust particles will make your hair tacky: try brushing it gently with a cologne-soaked cotton hanky over a brush once a day. Scratchy woolly hats won't ruin your hair-do if you line them with soft cotton or silk.

## Colouring your hair

Hair colourants are more subtle and safer to use than ever before. But if you tint your hair at home you must read the instructions and do a strand-test before you start.

Temporary colourants colour the surface of the hairshaft only and wash off with the next shampoo. Unless your hair is very porous through bleaching or sunbathing, there will be only a slight colour change.

Traditional semi-permanents penetrate the cuticle and deposit colour just inside the cortex of the hairshaft so that the natural and chemical colours mingle and last for about five to six shampoos. Red shades, dark browns and golden browns are successful on medium-brown and mousey hair.

Strong semi-permanents contain oxidation dyes like hydrogen peroxide which penetrate further into the cortex. Some

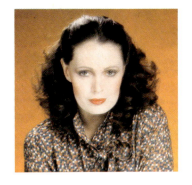

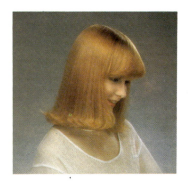

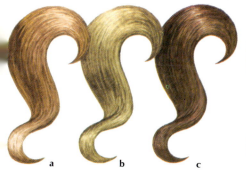

a      b      c

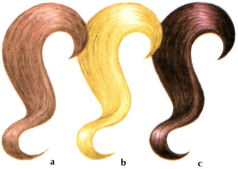

a      b      c

▲ *If you have naturally dark brown hair you can pick from all the red shades (a) including henna, but be guided by skin tone. A pale skin looks good with vibrant reds, a tawny skin with browny reds. Golden light brown (b) needs pre-lightening and toning and red highlights (c) involve an even longer process but look distinctively subtle.*

▲ *Naturally auburn hair goes with a pale skin and freckles, so take care: enhance your normal colour but don't change it completely. Bright red (a) will dramatize your looks and suit scarlet lipstick and clothes in creams and beiges. For golden red-blonde (b) pre-lighten and tone with golden blonde. Natural henna (c) will renew the hair's lustre, colour and body.*

shades could produce re-growth trouble, but most add colour which gradually washes out.

Permanent colourants are best used by the professionals. They penetrate the cortex with oxidation dyes which give complete colour change until it grows out.

Lighteners are mostly paired with a toner: the lightening agent strips pigment from the hairshaft, the toner adds it. A gentle lightener will lighten hair one to two shades, a medium lightener will go as far as four shades, and a 'maximum' product will go as far as you let it. These products also work more rapidly on porous hair. Never lighten your hair at home if your hair is in poor condition or has just been permed.

## Natural colouring agents

Natural colouring agents aren't always gentler than chemical-based ones. Henna, for instance, which coats the hairshaft and adds shine and body really works best on virgin dark hair or naturally red hair, but is less easy to control on tinted hair.

Lemon juice and camomile are good lightening agents for mousey or fair hair. Steep a tablespoonful of dried camomile flowers in a pint of boiling water, strain and cool and use as a rinse.

To add attractive highlights simply stroke half a cut lemon over your hair while you sunbathe, and to darken your hair try using sage leaves in place of camomile in the recipe above. Strong cold tea will also darken grey or mousey hair, as will an infusion of sage, marjoram and raspberry leaves.

## Perming

Perms are fabulous news for hair body and easy-care, but can be very bad news indeed for dry, out-of-condition or tinted hair. When hair is permed, the chemicals penetrate the hairshaft, and re-arrange the molecular structure of the hair which is then 'fixed' permanently by the neutralizing chemical. Your hair must be in good condition with no old perm, over-bleached ends, or other hair problems before your expensive perm.

Choose a style in a magazine to show your hairdresser before your perm and make sure you've picked the best hairdresser in your area. Allow yourself a whole afternoon or full Saturday morning because hurried perms look awful and you will definitely need a cut beforehand.

For home perms you need hair in good condition and a practical friend to succeed really well. You really can't go it alone unless you have very short hair and a lot of courage.

Permed styles look best washed, con-

**Blow-drying your hair**
This method of styling your hair gives soft shape, flicked-back sides and additional volume without the harder, more formal look of a roller set. But your hair should be expertly cut first and you must never overdry the hair by holding hairdryer too close.

1. Assemble equipment. Sit in front of a large mirror, towel-dry hair and pin top fringe and side hair on top of your head with long clips.

2. Working on the back hair first while you're fresh, hold the dryer in one hand and use the brush like a large roller in the other, curling the hair up from the roots and under as you dry.

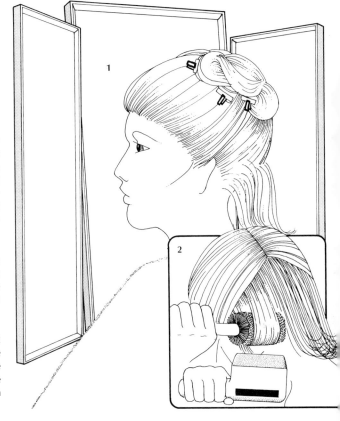

ditioned and left to dry naturally. They need not be brushed or combed, but you can set them on large rollers and dry your hair artificially. Try both methods. You can tint permed hair, but wait a week or two before tinting to allow the chemicals to settle. Perming after colouring will slightly lighten the colour.

## Common hair problems

Dandruff means a dry, flaky scalp and can be a problem whether hair is dry or greasy. Cut out rich, spicy foods and chocolate and drink extra water. Take yeast tablets and use a gentle medicated shampoo often.

Alopaecia or bald patches can be caused by hair abuse such as over-perming or heated rollers, which twist or harm the follicle itself, or it can be hormonal or hereditary. See a trichologist for professional help. The condition can occur after childbirth or if you stop taking the Pill. In these cases, the hair usually starts growing again quickly, provided your diet is good and you treat the hair gently.

Over-perming, hair abuse and illness can all contribute to damage your hair. For broken, split hair watch your diet and have your hair well cut regularly. No shampoo can 'mend' hair, although certain protein-based conditioners do penetrate the hair-shaft and help reconstruct damaged hair.

If you have greasy hair, eliminate fatty fried foods and sweets and cut down on oily foods. Use a gentle baby shampoo regularly.

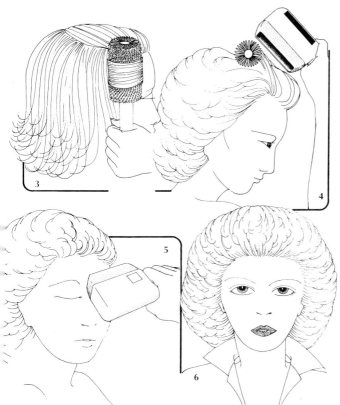

3. When the back section is complete, release the clips from the side hair and repeat the lifting and drying process. Brush hair back from the temples for the fashionable flicked-back look.

4. Now concentrate on the top of your hair-do, lifting each section at rightangles to the head and drying from the front.

5. Finally, the fringe and front hair. Your arms are probably quite tired by now, but keep up that lifting, rolling action. Now put the final touches to the sides of the hair-do.

6. Allow your hair to cool thoroughly before brushing gently into place. If it's a more casual style, you can lift and place the hair with your finger-tips.

# All about your skin

Skin is the body's protective covering; every two square centimetres (square inch) contains over 19 million cells, 65 hairs and muscles, around 100 sebaceous glands, 650 sweat glands, 78 nerves and 1,300 nerve endings that register pain. In addition, it registers heat, cold, touch, light and dark. To remain young-looking, skin needs water, for it is water that gives fresh, youthful skin its bloom, luminosity, softness and glow. Water helps build the cellular structure that makes up the three basic top layers: the epidermis, dermis and subdermis. It also helps maintain the protective acid mantle that covers the skin and fights off bacteria infection. In short, water is vital. Unfortunately, climatic conditions, central heating and the ageing process all rob the skin of water and, especially if the skin is dry in texture in the first place, this can lead to premature wrinkling, soreness and a dingy, unattractive look. Even if the skin is oily, water can *still* be in short supply.

Skin texture and appearance vary on different parts of the body. It's tougher on feet, hands, elbows, knees, softer on breasts, chest, neck, and softer still on nipples, lips, genital areas. Even on your face, the skin will appear very different in different areas. Your skin may be:

*Greasy:* on sides of your nose, chin and around your mouth. Pores may be enlarged, with the sebaceous glands pumping out sebum, which combines with sweat and

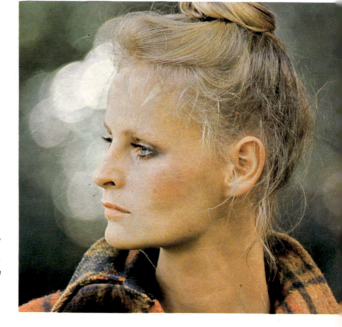

▶ Healthy skin has a clear, blemish-free texture and a slightly luminous quality. Although make-up can help disguise imperfections, it can't hide blemishes or dryness completely. So, aim to get your skin into the best possible condition. Start naturally, by watching your diet. Eat plenty of fresh fruit, salads and dairy products. Give your skin regular daily care and, above all, treat it gently.

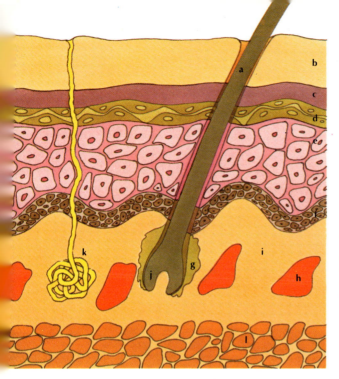

◀ Here's a greatly enlarged cross-section of human skin showing the top two layers, the epidermis and the dermis.

(a) hair shaft
(b) stratum corneum, the horny layer, consists of closely packed keratin (protein) cells which rub off and are renewed from the stratum germinativum.
(c) stratum lucidum
(d) stratum granulosum
(e) stratum mucosum
(f) stratum germinativum
(g) sebaceous glands which release sebum to give the skin softness and bloom. In puberty sebaceous glands can be over-active, causing a sebum build-up leading to spots and acne.
(h) blood vessels
(i) dermis
(j) papilla
(k) perspiration gland and duct
(l) fatty tissue

debris to block the pores and produce spots, pimples and pustules. Maybe the greasiness extends to other facial areas too, although this is unusual in Northern Europeans, apart from during puberty.

*Dry:* with flakiness, tiny lines around eyes, mouth, and sore spots on cheekbones. It probably 'drinks in' creams and lotions, feels dry after bathing.

*Sensitive:* it may be dry, greasy, or a combination of both. It becomes irritated or sore when rubbed or when harsh products are used, reacts with rashes, sore spots or blotches in sun or bad weather, itches if you wear fluffy sweaters, scarves, tight collars.

## How to care for your skin

*Greasy:* watch your diet. Exclude greasy, fried foods, add extra vitamin C (oranges), drink water. Wash greasy areas with bland soap or clean with liquid-based cleanser. Use gentle, non-oily moisturizer, water-based foundation.

*Dry:* add vegetable oils to your diet, and vitamin C. Cleanse skin with moisturized cleanser (*not* soap), use creamy foundation, moisturize morning and night. Use rich, light cream on eye areas (apply with fingertips and patting action). Give neck regular nourishing beauty mask treatment.

*Sensitive:* use bland preparations as your skin may react badly to perfume and alcohol, and cleanse lightly with liquid cleanser. Hypo-allergenic moisturizers and foundations do 'screen out' many of the potentially irritating substances, but often even more harm is done to a delicate skin by bad hygiene than by the cosmetics themselves. Be scrupulously careful about washing hands, make-up brushes, face flannel, comb, brush and make-up bag.

# Are you allergic to these cosmetic ingredients?

Here's a list of known allergens commonly used in beauty products which could cause trouble. If you suspect that you are allergic to one or more of these then try switching to a hypo-allergenic brand of make-up which excludes the villain. If you want to know precisely what is in a particular product and it isn't marked on the package, then contact the manufacturer for advice. Note: sometimes you can quite suddenly become sensitive to an ingredient that has lived happily on your skin for years! Dermatologists sometimes have to carry out many patch tests before they are able to track down the precise cause of an allergy. If you have *any* persistent rash or itching symptoms, do contact your doctor for advice.

| COSMETIC GROUP | SUBSTANCES | SYMPTOMS |
|---|---|---|
| **Skin care and perfume products** | Almond oil (creams, lotions, perfumes) | Rhinitis, dermatitis venenata |
| | Alcohol (fresheners, astringents, perfumes) | Dermatitis venenata, excessive dryness |
| | Balsam of peru (perfumes) | Rhinitis, dermatitis venenata, hayfever |
| | Benhaldehyde (creams, lotions) | Dermatitis venenata |
| | Lanoline (creams, lotions) | Dermatitis venenata |
| | Methyl heptine carbonate (perfumes, toilet waters, perfumed cosmetics) | Dermatitis venenata, hayfever, asthma, dermatitis, photosensitivity |
| | Zinc chloride, zinc sulphate (astringent lotions) | Dermatitis venenata |
| **Lipsticks** | Dibrom and tetrabram-fluorescein (gives staining effect of indelible lipsticks) | Lip inflammation, tummy upsets |
| | Perfume and flavouring oils (in lip gloss) | Inflammation, hayfever, asthma, dermatitis, photosensitivity |
| **Powders and blushers** | Cornstarch (face powders, blushers and body talcs) | Conjunctivitis, rhinitis, hayfever |
| | Wheatstarch, gum tragacanth (compacts) | Catarrh, dermatitis, tummy upset |
| **Nail varnish and remover** | Acetone (remover) | Peeling and splitting nails, dermatitis of fingers, face, eyes |
| | Sulfonamide resins (varnish) | Itching on nails, eyelids, face or body, dermatitis venenata |
| **Body care** | Almond oil (soap) | Rhinitis, dermatitis venenata |
| | Aluminium salts (deodorants) | Dermatitis venenata, rhinitis, conjunctivitis |

*All skin types*: protect your skin from cold, dirt, wind and rain with a good moisturizer, even if you don't wear make-up all the time. Remember to extend skin care to your throat, since this area often gets neglected. Always treat your skin gently and beware of harsh products, like strong astringents which could make your skin over-dry and sore.

## Your summer skin

A suntan is sexy, attractive, rich-looking, but it can be disastrous for your skin. There is no doubt that the sun dries and ages all skin types. That's why it's vital to protect your skin against the harmful short ultra-violet rays that burn as well as tan. Most sensitive are skins that contain little melanin, the substance that actually produces the brown pigment in your skin. Blondes, redheads and Celtic types have less melanin than dark-haired people and must therefore be especially careful in the sun. The most vulnerable ages for burning are, for children, from 6-8; for women, from 25-30 and for men, from 30-35.

If you decide you want a glowing suntan, plan your tanning campaign before you go on holiday. Step up the vitamin A foods in your diet (carrots, apricots, butter, eggs) and prepare your skin with daily lubricant rubs with baby oil or body lotion. Use a tanning lotion containing bergamot oil to soak up some of the weaker sunshine before you go to hotter climates. This substance helps you get a tan even in the park at lunchtime. Or, take a series of ultra-violet tanning treatments at a beauty salon to encourage melanin to protect your skin and take the agony out of the first few days in the sun.

Aim for a tan which suits your skin type or just be pale and interesting if the whole process is a painful bore. Arm yourself with a light voile long-sleeved dress and a shady hat and swim when the sun is lowest in the morning or evening. Tans became fashionable for their rarity-value: the 'gilded lily' look is now *much* more rare.

Fake tanning preparations give a convincing tan, but can be tricky to apply. The best way is to use them after a bath when you have applied a body lotion all over. Work the fake tan upwards from your toes in even, sweeping movements. Rub well in. Blot porous skin areas such as knees and elbows with tissue and wash your hands thoroughly. Stay naked for 15-30 minutes, to allow the lotion to sink into your skin befor putting on your clothes. Fake tanning lotions or tinted make-ups are useful for your face: baking accelerates wrinkles, and produces peeling nose, sore lips and headaches. Fake it, and wear a hat. Here's a guide to the tanning lotions to choose, according to your skin-type. Most these days contain para-aminobenzoic acid combined with softeners and lubricants. One range contains guanin, a DA factor which provides protection to the skin cells *beneath* the surface of the skin: this gives a very efficient protective treatment indeed.

## Fair, very sensitive skin

Don't try to beat nature. Stay cool and pale by swimming in the early morning or late evening, sitting in the shade during the hot mid-day hours. Use a sun-block to screen out the UV rays on your most sensitive areas: nose, breasts, feet, thighs. When swimming, use a water-resistant, water-in-oil formula sun lotion to prevent burning.

## Sensitive skin, burns easily

Use a sun-block on sensitive areas, a lotion with a high protective factor (5,6) at first, then a lower factor (3) when you start to get brown. Allow yourself a five-minute sun-bathe only on day one, ten minutes on day three and increase to a maximum of 30

▼ *A golden summer skin will flatter any figure and complexion and can now be acquired in a matter of minutes thanks to the wide range of reliable fake tanning lotions available. If you still prefer the traditional way of turning brown, do it safely and follow the dos and don'ts in this chapter.*

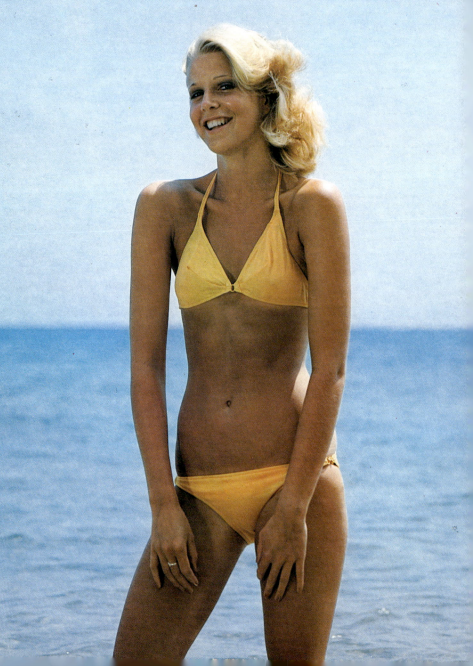

minutes on day 14. A course of six ultra-violet sessions before your holiday would save time and agony!

## Normal skin, burns sometimes

Use a high-protective cream on sensitive areas, a waterproof lotion when swimming or sailing. Switch to oil when your tan becomes established. Start with a ten-minute sunbathe, morning and evening, gradually increasing to three 30-minute sessions. *Never* mid-day.

## Olive skin, tans easily

Use an oil, but smooth on high-protective cream if you expose new areas to the sun—nipples, for instance. Start with a 20-minute morning and evening sunbathe and increase to four 30-minute sessions. *Not* mid-day.

## All skin-types

Use après-sun lotion after your evening shower. Apply cold tea to sensitive spots. To make your tan last longer, add baby oil to your bathwater, avoid scratchy clothes, don't scrub your skin hard. Tan tip: those 'pinky' bits turn brown overnight if you use a fake tanning lotion on them before bedtime.

## Suntan factors

Many suntan products carry suntan factors on the packet. The higher numbers (5, 6, 7) give the best protection against the danger-ous short ultra-violet rays. They are suitable for sensitive skins in northern European countries and all skins in southern European countries. Use the highest number (7) if you go skiing, as the thin atmosphere at high altitudes makes the effect of the sun more fierce. The lower numbers (2, 3, 4) are suitable for normal skins in northern Europe and are fine once your tan is established.

## The sun and ageing

As well as following a sensible tan plan, make sure that you cover your head with a shady hat and invest in some good anti-glare glasses. Deep wrinkles are often permanently formed around the eyes when skin has been puckered by squinting and dried out by high temperatures.

After swimming, make sure you rinse the salt water from your body and face, and remember that although the wind and water don't intensify the sun's rays, they do make you feel cooler, and therefore less alert to potential harm.

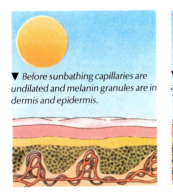

▼ *Before sunbathing capillaries are undilated and melanin granules are in dermis and epidermis.*

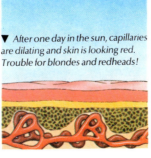

▼ *After one day in the sun, capillaries are dilating and skin is looking red. Trouble for blondes and redheads!*

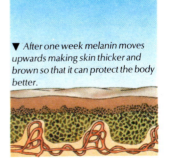

▼ *After one week melanin moves upwards making skin thicker and brown so that it can protect the body better.*

# Look after your teeth

Healthy teeth are a beauty asset that, sadly, is becoming increasingly rare. Dental disease is the commonest disease of mankind: over eight million teeth are extracted in Britain alone each year. Now the dental profession is putting much more emphasis on preventative work to try and cut down the problems of dental caries (decay) and peridontal disorders such as gingivitis (gum disease). Many dentists even have full or part-time dental hygienists who specialize in helping patients to correct tooth, gum and general mouth-care techniques.

As well as using these dental services by making sure you get a check-up every six months there is a great deal you can do at home to keep your teeth healthy. It really isn't enough to brush them casually twice a day with a worn-out toothbrush and hope for the best! You need to understand the underlying causes of dental disorders first and how to combat them.

Plaque is the breeding-ground for most tooth and gum troubles. This is the thin invisible film which is constantly being formed on the teeth. It contains food debris, bacteria and saliva and is the root cause of many very big problems. It must be completely removed at least twice a day. If you think you do a pretty good brushing job already, then try an experiment with 'disclosing' tablets from your chemist. These, dissolved in water and swished around your mouth produce a bright red stain that clings solely to plaque and can easily be brushed clean. Usually, you'll find that plaque deposits remain between your teeth and clinging to the crevices around the gums even if you've conscientiously brushed your teeth just before using the tablets. This is because most people just don't brush

between their teeth. Unless you use dent floss (a wax-covered twine available fror chemists) or invest in a special interspac toothbrush with a rounded head to searc out food debris between your teeth, yo won't get rid of plaque.

Floss is easy to use: you simply wind the twine around your two forefingers and push the taut twine between your teeth making sawing movement to remove all food debris Do this all around your mouth—back a well as front teeth. Rinse thoroughly, ther

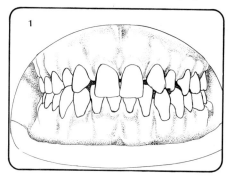

*1. The patient's teeth have an unfortunate vampire-like appearance.*

concentrate on brushing: brush the back teeth which actually grind the food particles and work all around the front teeth in an up-and-down movement. Rinse again.

Don't expect your toothbrush to last more than four months at the outside. Choose a brush with a maximum number of non-scratchy bristles or tufts on the head; they should be flexible, round-ended, pliable. Although it's been shown that fluoride-containing toothpastes do help reduce fillings, especially in children, you should rely on your own thorough brushing rather than the toothpaste, and beware of abrasive

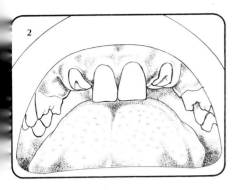

2. They are prepared for crowning by cutting them back and drilling holes in them. Temporary teeth are inserted while the gold crown pegs and porcelain crowns are being prepared.

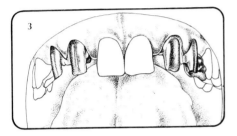

3. The pegs are fitted into the prepared holes. Gold is used for its strength and mouldability in dental work, which accounts for the expense of the operation.

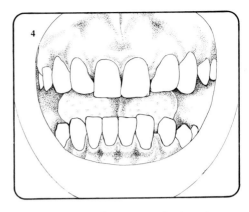

4. The finished porcelain crowns are fitted over the pegs. The patient can smile with confidence!

## Cosmetic dentistry

Many bad dental problems can be helped by the exciting new techniques of cosmetic dentistry. More and more dentists are working in this field, and your own dentist is probably much more willing to crown, cap or bridge your teeth than he was, say, five years ago. If you're in danger of losing a tooth, do explore all the cosmetic possibilities first. They may be expensive, but in many cases the cost is worthwhile.

Crowns are artificial teeth, carefully matched to your own, which are fixed to gold pins inserted into the root of your tooth stump. The fixing involves several visits to the dentist and can be painful. Temporary crowns are usually put in place while the 'custom-made' ones are carefully made. Crowns are useful where teeth are badly out of line, uneven, broken, or eroded by grinding on acidic foods.

Bridgework involves inserting one or more teeth into a gap by suspending the 'falsies' on a bridge from crowns on two adjoining teeth. If you lose one or more teeth in an accident or by bad caries or gum disorders, bridgework can save you from the problems and inconvenience of a plate with the false teeth attached.

smokers' toothpaste which could remove the enamel on your teeth as well as the yellow stains! For the same reason, limit your intake of very acidic drinks: dentists now favour ending a meal with a bland food such as cheese instead of the traditional apple, to leave the mouth in a non-acidic state.

Diet generally is vitally important if you are to avoid caries. Keep off sticky, gooey foods, especially when there is no opportunity to clean your teeth after you've eaten them. Always make sure you have plenty of water to drink after meals and brush your teeth at work or if you're out; it's simple to tuck a toothbrush and a small tube of paste in your bag or pocket.

# Care for your hands

Hands are often a neglected area, beauty-wise, which is a pity, for smooth hands and well manicured nails are a great morale-booster. You really don't have to spend a great deal of time on caring for your hands if you do just three things: give yourself a

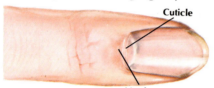

**Cuticle**

**Matrix**

manicure once a week (see below); put handcream in strategic places where you'll use it, like by the sink; and wear rubber gloves for tough chores. If you follow these rules, you'll only need to reapply an extra coat of polish once or twice a week to keep your hands in tip-top shape.

Nails can be a problem, and some of the products on the market are not as effective as the manufacturers claim. Nails are made from closely-packed cells of keratin, a

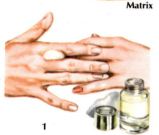

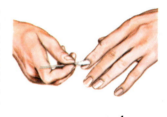

1. You need: cotton wool; varnish and remover; orange sticks; emery boards; hand cream; cuticle remover; top coat. Start by removing old varnish: hold cotton wool between first and second fingers and rub nails against it rather than the other way around.

2. Now file nails gently away from you; make a smooth oval shape, and don't file away too much nail at the sides, or the nails will snap more easily and could develop hang-nails and soreness. Emery boards are less harsh than metal nail files.

3. Use the pointed end of an orange stick plus a little bit of cotton wool, to clean away any dirt or debris under the nail. A little cuticle remover on the cotton wool will help clean the area thoroughly.

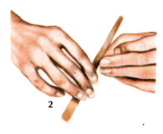

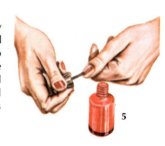

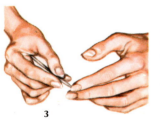

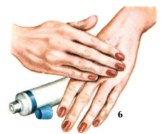

protein, which grows from the matrix area. Good nutrition (see p. 6-11) is the first essential for strong nails. If they become brittle with longitudinal ridging, this could mean you're suffering from mild anaemia. If you have white spots, make sure you're getting enough vitamin A from carrots, liver and fish oils. Flaky nails mean your nail polish or remover may be too harsh: switch to a cream enamel as the pearly ones are more likely to cause flaking and use plenty of conditioning oil during your manicure.

Tough nail enamels sometimes don't last any longer than ordinary enamels. Nail conditioners containing protein won't perform miracles since the amount contained in the formula will only soften the nail and surrounding skin. Look after your nails if you want them to grow long: an average growth-rate is six months from root to tip!

To give your nails the treatment, try filling a used half-lemon with olive or corn oil. Leave overnight, then use the lotion as a nail and hand-softener. Lemon peel will help strengthen nails if you rub it on during your manicure. Lemon helps restore the skin's own natural acid-balance, a protective mantle which is often destroyed by alkaline soaps and household chemicals.

▼ *Red or rust-coloured nail enamels go with most clothes, and look stunningly glamorous, but you must watch out for chipping.*

4. Apply tiny blobs of cuticle remover or cream to each cuticle. Smooth in very gently. Now, using the wedge-end of the orange stick, ease back the cuticle and remove any stray bits of skin which come away, until the halfmoon (which is really the top of the matrix or growth area of the nail) is revealed.

5. Apply a little extra remover to each nail to get rid of greasiness before the varnish is applied. Painting the nails on your right hand first, make three strokes on each nail: centre, left side, right side, working from halfmoon towards the tip.

6. Allow nails 10 minutes to dry before reapplying varnish. Dark enamels usually need only two coats; lighter shades need three. Apply a top-coat of clear gloss for extra shine and protection. Now pamper your hands with handcream.

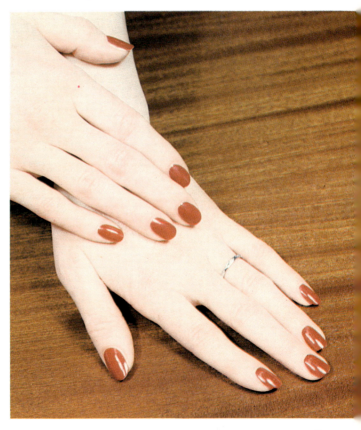

# Foot care

Beautiful feet are an obvious asset in summer, but in winter, too, they are vital for good looks. If your feet hurt it shows—on your *face!* Make sure your shoes and boots leave plenty of room for toes to wiggle freely, and the heel-height allows comfortable walking. Aim for support under and over the arch of the foot: a good heel-grip and fairly high-cut sides or an instep strap.

Watch out for these foot problems which should be treated by your doctor or chiropodist:

1. Corns and callouses are caused by friction, the callous being a flatter form of corn.

2. Verrucae are painful brownish spots caused by a fungus infection commonly found in warm, damp places such as

Boots can be the cause of lasting foot problems if they are (a) too tight round the calf, restricting circulation; (b) chafing the heel, causing blisters and hard skin; (c) pinching the toe, causing foot deformities and corns.

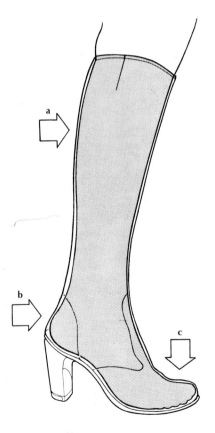

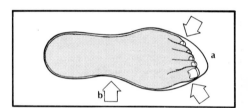

Shoes can damage the feet if they are (a) too pointed, causing involuted nails, bone deformities, corns and bunions; (b) there is inadequate support around the instep so the foot slides forward and presses on the front of the shoe (c), causing hammer toes, corns and nail deformities.

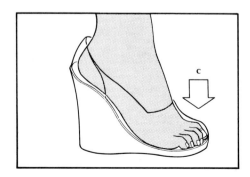

wimming baths and gyms.

3. Athlete's foot is also a fungus-type infection, which thrives in damp, warm conditions. It feels itchy and is irritated by woolly socks, soft shoes.

4. In-growing toenails are usually preceded by inflamed skin and caused by bad trimming. Never try to treat this condition yourself.

5. Bunions are missaligned joints which become swollen and tender inside ill-fitting shoes. Although the condition may be hereditary, good shoes certainly help.

6. Involuted nails (usually on big toes only) grow inwards from the matrix or nail bed. Often caused by missaligned nail regrowth when the original nail has been lost, they can be successfully treated with a minor operation.

Take time for a weekly foot-pampering treatment. Follow the instructions for the manicure on p. 56 but separate toes with cotton wool balls for easier handling. Always clip or trim nails straight across.

A good natural skin-softener for your feet is olive oil. In summer, sprinkle talc into your shoes and wash tights in lavender-scented water or go barefoot. When you wash your feet, add a teaspoonful of cider vinegar to the water for a refreshing, deodorizing rinse. Don't use hot water: this destroys the natural skin-softeners, dilates the blood vessels and could make feet sore and more prone to chafing.

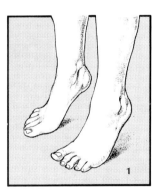

1. To strengthen toes and arches take off your shoes and walk on tip-toes for a few moments. Now raise up and lower alternate feet on tip-toes 50 times. Good for tired feet.

2. To strengthen feet and ankles sit on a chair, feet on the floor. Roll feet outwards, toes together. Hold position and return 30 times.

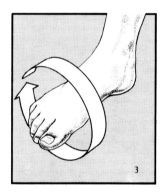

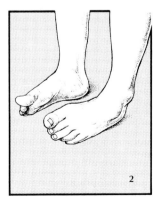

3. To slim and strengthen ankles, sit on a chair and rotate feet clockwise 20 times, then anti-clockwise.

4. To increase suppleness, strengthen toes, pick up a pencil with your toes, 10 times for each foot.

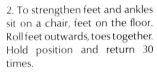

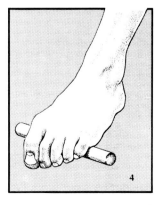

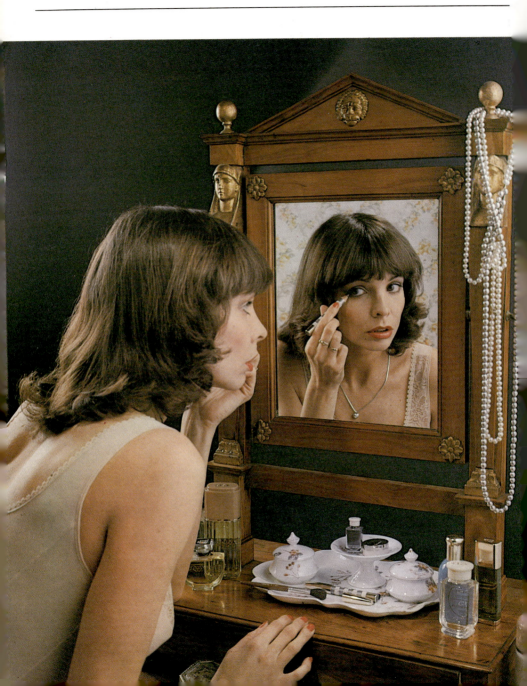

Make-up techniques have never been as exciting and effective as they are today, and products have never been as numerous. It's easy to become confused and even indignant about the huge ranges of often-unnecessary, badly-packaged 'beauty aids' on the market. Keep a cool head, be selective and you can look beautifully made-up whatever your face-shape, skin-type or faults may be.

*Your top priority should be the tools of the trade.* Buy good-quality brushes and cosmetic sponges; a headband to wear while you put on your face; soft tissues or cotton wool for removing make-up; non-scratchy tweezers for eyebrow plucking; and a pencil sharpener with two holes for fat and thin cosmetic pencils.

Keep your equipment where you can see exactly what you've got. A knife-drawer lined with pretty washable wallpaper is ideal: tuck it out of sight into the top drawer of your dressing table. Arrange eye shadows in one compartment (take them out of the box), lip-colour in another, blushers and foundation in another. Use a conventional make-up bag simply to transport lip-colour, mirror and mascara inside your handbag. Have regular 'weeding out' sessions where you ruthlessly discard old make-up.

Cut the cost of looking good by using refills where possible (pretty packaging accounts for 90 per cent of the cost of some products). If you want to try a new colour, buy the smallest, cheapest version first or cadge a free trial from the cosmetic counter. Most liquid foundations are best applied with a wet sponge, and this cuts down the amount you actually use. Eye make-up remover pads can be made to last twice as long if you sandwich them between circles of lint in the box. Lip colour is best applied with a brush and lasts much longer than when stroked on from the stick.

Be prepared to experiment—it's often a good way of saving money. For instance,

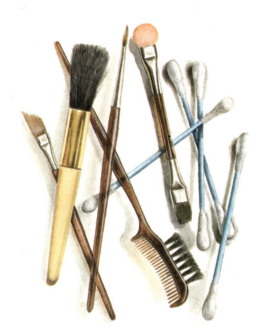

▲ *Brushes for beauty, left to right : wedge-shaped brush for lipstick ; large, soft rouge-mop brush for blusher ; finely pointed eye-liner brush ; eye-brow comb with built-in brush for separating lashes after applying mascara ; double-ended sponge and eyeshadow brush ; cotton wool buds.*

many glossy lip 'wands' can be used as blusher; blushers can double as eye colour; kohl eye contour pencils can be used for brows too.

## Your make-up in easy stages

Start with a prepared 'canvas'; smooth a light moisturizer all over your face and neck and let it sink in for a few moments. This will soften and protect your skin.

Apply a light, beige-tinted foundation with a cosmetic sponge. This tone suits most skins, but if you have an olive-toned skin, choose a honey shade. Beware of pinky-tinted foundations: they look dated. Add

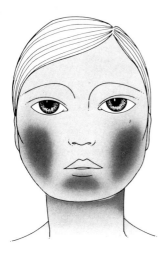

◀ *Soften the corners of a square face with tawny shader on lower cheeks and temples. Highlight the tops of your cheekbones and your chin.*

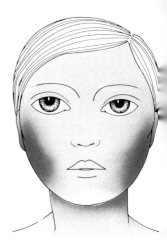

▶ *Give a round face interesting angles by using shader on your cheeks in upwards strokes towards ear-level. Add highlighter to chin. Blend all 'edges'.*

any colour to this base later on. Apply the foundation in downwards strokes, to smooth out the hairs on your face, but don't put any on your eyelids because foundations are creamy and could make your eye colour 'melt' into tiny lines. Take the foundation down under the chin and blend it into your neck, but not down to collar-level.

Apply powder hygienically with cotton wool and use a translucent, no-colour powder for a pearly, sheeny look. Press well into skin, then brush off the surplus with fresh cotton wool or a baby brush.

## Blusher, highlighter, shader

Apply powder highlighter, blusher and shader using the face-shapes above as a guide to position. Remember that they must be subtle: blend in all 'edges' and use a very light touch with your rouge 'mop' brush. In summer, try using a creamy blusher high on your cheekbones over foundation only and no powder. This gives a gleaming, glowing look. Experiment with blushers: earlobes, chin and temples sometimes look good with a tawny or pinkish glow. Avoid dark or blue-red shades and stick to peach, light rust and tawny colours for the best results.

## Eyes

First use a water-based creamy-coloured eye shade all over the lid and up to the browbone as a foundation. Next, choose the colours you need. Best for blondes are greys, browns, beiges, greens and pinky-peach colours. Browns, beiges, blue-greys, greens and rusts suit brunettes, and red-heads should choose browns, greens, blues, rust, violets and pinky-peach colours. Follow the guide on p. 55 for correcting eye shape faults and be prepared to use three or more colours, blending them in very carefully. Powder colours are easiest to control, but the wand-type stay put quite well if you blend them in with a brush afterwards. Creamy gloss colours invariably crease so avoid them unless you want a very glossy look for a party.

Eye make-up dates more quickly than anything else, so follow magazine features for the latest ideas. Remember: subtle colours look more professional and you can often achieve effective results from kohl, the

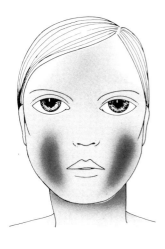

◀ *A little dark shading under your chin and around your jawline will shorten an oblong face, and you can use highlighter on your temples to give a flattering lift.*

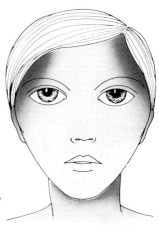

▶ *Plump out the cheeks of a heart-shaped face with rosy blusher and use a tawny shader to soften the temples and prevent a 'triangular' look from spoiling a good shape.*

soft eye pencil that is used around the inner rim of the eye. Apply it before mascara like this: gently pull lower lid down, and trace a fine line with a soft, sharp kohl pencil along the inner rim. Blink a few times. Apply to upper inner eye rim. Blink again. Don't use it if you have sensitive, bloodshot eyes. Now apply mascara, upwards on upper lashes, downwards on lower. Use non-filament mascaras which are easy to clean off: long-lasting mascaras will make removal difficult and thin out your lashes. Three coats, with careful brushing between will give a natural, fluttery look.

## Brows

Brush brows upwards into a neat line and pluck out any stragglers underneath the natural shape, stretching the skin with the first and second fingers of the left hand, while you pluck with the tweezers held firmly in the right. A natural look is high fashion now, so don't overdo it. If necessary, darken brows like this: brush hairs towards the nose, pencil in light, feathery strokes to correct and darken the brow, using a sharp pencil in grey/brown or brown/black (not

black). Now brush brows upwards and outwards to cover and soften the pencilled strokes.

## Lips

Lip shape and colour is a vital part of the fashion look. First, apply foundation all over your lips. Now, using a sharp pinky-brown lip pencil, trace the outline of your lip shape. Correct your lip-line like this: if your lips are narrow, make the line outside your natural shape. If they are too full, make it inside the natural shape. Lop-sided lips can also be corrected at this stage. It's fashionable to draw a fairly pointed 'cupid's bow' on the upper lip, but don't exaggerate this too much. Fill in with colour from a lipstick, gloss-pot or wand, but whichever you choose, apply it with a brush, blot on tissue then reapply. Remember, the creamier and glossier the colour, the less stable it will be. Often lips look best if you use a conventional cream-formula lipstick with a clear gloss on top. This method is less likely to leave a nasty, sticky residue on your teeth, teacups, cigarettes, collars etc! As for colour, red and tawny are glamorous; pink more subtle.

## How to be quick on the draw

With pencils you can achieve dazzling beauty effects, if you know how.

First, buy soft, creamy eye, cheek and lip pencils and keep them sharp. If they crumble easily pop them in the fridge for half an hour before sharpening. If they are too hard, soften the colour by rubbing the pencil in a little moisturizer in your hand, especially before applying to eyes.

Double-ended pencils are usually colour-toned for subtle eye make-up: look for rust cream shades for eyes and lips; silver and pewter shades for sparkly party eyes; forest and willow-green shades to use around brown/blue or hazel eyes for a wide-eyed autumn look.

Pencils have other advantages: they're spill-proof and take up little room in your

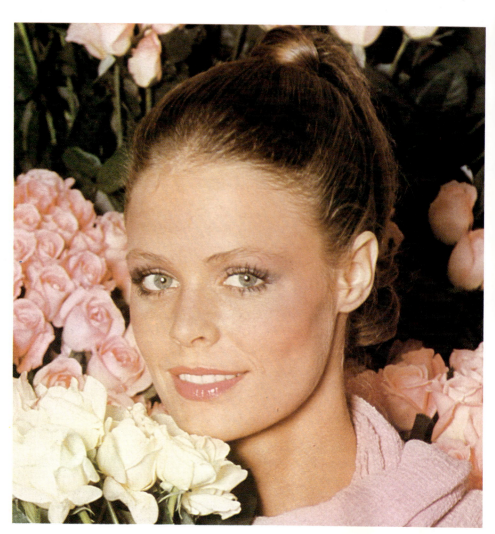

bag. Try using just one pencil for your entire beach make-up; tawny peach for lips, blusher, eye-colour worn over a suntan lotion or moisturizing lotion. Add mascara, a mirror and a pencil sharpener, and you've got a complete beauty kit. Three double-ended pencils would give you a colour wardrobe for an entire season. You can also blend colours together using the moisturizer-in-your-hand softening method above and applying the mixture with a soft brush.

A magnifying mirror on a stand helps accurate application, as does an elbow on your table or dressing-table as you work. Look *down* into the glass when using eye colour to expose your entire lid area. Never wet a pencil in your mouth, as eye irritations can be started very quickly indeed by bacteria.

## It's all done with pencils

Here's a beautiful, subtle make-up which has been applied with just three basic tools, a soft black pencil and two pens in peachy pink for eyes and blusher and cherry pink for lips. The foundation is a basic sunshine-beige, blended right under the chin. Next, the peachy pen was applied very lightly to the eyelids, extending outwards and slightly under the eye. Then, the mouth was outlined with the cherry pen and filled in very lightly —blotted with tissue and re-applied. The peachy pen was used on the cheekbones as a subtle blusher. The soft but sharp black velvet pencil was used on the inner rim of the eye. Finally, brownish-black mascara was used in three coats.

◄ *This entire look, bar the mascara, has been achieved with three pencils. With this method you can save on space, time and money and look simply beautiful.*

**Before make-up**          **After make-up**

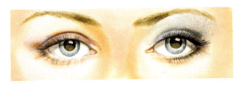

▲ *Are your eyes too close? Make them appear wide apart by using pale shadow on the inner corners, a 'wing' of darker shadow from the centre lid upwards and outwards. Kohl on outer rim only.*

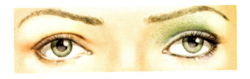

▲ *Too wide apart? Use darker shadow on the inner corners and shade from inner socket outwards, stopping at the natural outer corner of each eye.*

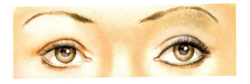

▲ *Too small? Open up the eye area with light shadow around the eye, soft brown kohl lines around the eye rim, beige/brown wings of shadow from socket to brow-bone.*

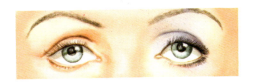

▲ *If your eyes are hooded, dark shadow will make the lid appear smaller. Blend it into a lighter shadow on the brow-bone. Use more light shadow under the eye area.*

# Disguising problem areas

Make-up is marvellously versatile and it can effectively disguise many facial imperfections. Even severe problems like strawberry birthmarks can be camouflaged if you know how. But, if possible it's always a good idea to get special advice from a beautician for specific problems—and a make-up lesson on handling and concealing them. Many top beauticians are specially trained in the art of cosmetic disguise; there is no need to feel embarrassed about contacting your local beauty salon or a cosmetic manufacturer for specific advice, and this applies to men, as well as women.

**Dark circles** If early nights, compresses and soothing lotions still leave you with dark circles under your eyes, then disguise them like this: after using moisturizer, but before putting on your foundation, apply a very pale creamy disguising base to the area with a brush. These bases usually come in stick-form: it's best to soften them in moisturizer in your hand, then dab on carefully. Top with beige foundation pressed onto your skin with a sponge.

**Flushes** Excitement, the menopause, tension can all produce embarrassing flushes on face, neck and chest. Use a green-based moisturizer on the problem area, topped by a pale foundation and a thick coating of translucent powder applied with cotton wool. Brush off surplus and set the disguise with a cold flannel, very lightly applied. *Don't* spray perfume on the area, it could irritate it. Avoid alcohol.

**Birthmarks** Use stick make-up, of the theatrical kind. Apply with a brush, blending in with the surrounding skin-tone. The darker the mark, the paler the make-up should be. Now top the make-up, if necessary, with a foundation that tones with the surrounding facial skin, and continue the make-up all over the face. Set with translucent powder.

**Wrinkles** Powder makes wrinkles look deeper, skin look older, so instead, smooth on a liquid make-up with a sponge dipped in water, using a very light touch indeed on wrinkled areas like neck, forehead, eyes, lids. Use a water-spray during the day to freshen your face and reduce creases.

**Thread veins** Nose area and cheeks are the most common spots for this problem. Always use a rich moisturizer as cold weather or sunshine makes them more pronounced and top it with beige foundation mixed with pale disguise stick make-up in your hand and applied with a brush. Loose powder looks too dry and flaky on this kind of fine skin, so press on creamy compressed powder with a damp sponge instead.

**Receding chin** Bring your chin forward by using a foundation one shade lighter than on the rest of your face. Blend in the joins with a brush. Hair bounce on the crown of your head helps too.

**Bags** Don't be tempted to powder over bags under your eyes, but apply one coat of foundation in a beige shade with a damp sponge instead. Use extra eye colour above your eyes (none underneath) and put a little blusher on your temples. This will successfully draw attention to the top half of your face.

**Acne scars** Pale liquid foundation, dabbed on with a sponge topped by powder pressed on with cotton wool, is the best disguise for these scars. Dermabrasion operations are worth considering.

**Big nose** Shade sides and tip of nose with browny-beige shader and make a narrow

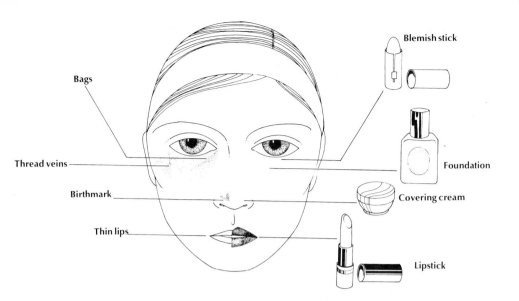

Bags

Thread veins

Birthmark

Thin lips

Blemish stick

Foundation

Covering cream

Lipstick

▲ *Above, a basically good skin is marred by blemishes. Disguise bags under the eyes with a blemish-stick;* *thread veins with a green-based foundation; birthmarks with covering cream. Then apply a liquid foundation* *in beige to the whole face and top with translucent powder applied with cotton wool. Brush off surplus.*

line of gleaming highlighter—try eye shadows, applied with a brush—down the bridge, ending before the natural tip of your nose. This line will pick up the light and give the illusion of a short, stylish nose!

**Double chin** Use darker foundation under the chin, blending downwards very carefully indeed. Keep your chin up!

**High forehead** Blusher on temples gives a warm glow. Shade beige foundation to a slightly darker tint near the hair line. Keep hair soft on your forehead, and darken your brows if they are pale, to avoid a 'medieval' look.

**Shiny areas** Use a non-oily base over light moisturizer which you've allowed to sink in first. Powder lightly, 'set' with a wet flannel, and leave alone. Don't be tempted to re-powder every few hours, or you'll end up with a thick, gooey mess and blocked pores.

**Large ears** Disguise large lobes with dark foundation, cover entire ear with medium-toned foundation and translucent powder. Wear your hair over your ears in soft waves or a chic long bob cut.

**Unwanted hair** Pluck out or disguise a light growth with a mild solution of bleach applied with cotton wool. Otherwise, have them removed permanently with electrolysis.

**Warts and moles** A light touch disguises these: use a stick covering make-up, with a very fine brush. Stroke just a little make-up over the blemish, and blend in before applying foundation on the rest of your face. Do seek advice about removing warts and moles professionally.

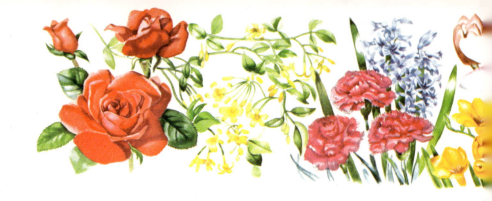

# You and your fragrance

Nothing creates a beautiful mood more perfectly than the right fragrance. Perfume is an integral part of the beauty scene, the very essence of style, atmosphere, memory.

Most perfumes are blended by 'noses' who work for one of the ten top essential essence houses. The formula is then sold to the fashion organization or the cosmetic company. Most, with the exception of a very few, like Chanel, don't do their own blending. This is because the art of perfumery is a subtle and complicated one— indeed there are only about 35 'noses' in the world! These experts can recognize the subtle 'notes' of different essential oils and can 'orchestrate' them into new, original perfumes. They are trained at the world's perfume essence centre in Grasse, Provence, France, where the oils are distilled, stored and distributed.

Ingredients include a blend of floral and herbal oils, like rose, jasmine, hyacinth, lily of the valley, camomile, mint and sage, spices such as coriander and woody fragrances such as sandalwood. The perfume may have several 'notes': the first impact-making smell, followed by the deeper, more heady fragrance, then perhaps an even richer fragrance when the formula has mixed and blended with the natural body smells.

Cheaper perfumes usually have fewer subtle 'notes' and less lasting-power than the more expensive, classic perfumes, but many are excellent value if you want glamour at a lower price and are happy to re-use them often throughout the day.

When choosing scent, the most important consideration is whether you adore the smell. This seems obvious, but with so many advertised 'images' to choose from, you could be more influenced by the girl or man on the package than the perfume itself! Try out several perfumes at a time from the testers provided by the stores, using these ingredients as a guide to your type, although you shouldn't take it as a rigid ruling.

## Your type, your fragrance

1. Light, floral and citrus scents including lemon, bergamot, hyacinth, scented mosses, honeysuckle and iris are good for sporty types, young people, people who work with others.

2. Musky, leathery scents including musk, myrrh, spices like coriander, heavy florals like patchouli, and jasmine take a lot of living up to! Use them for evening or day-

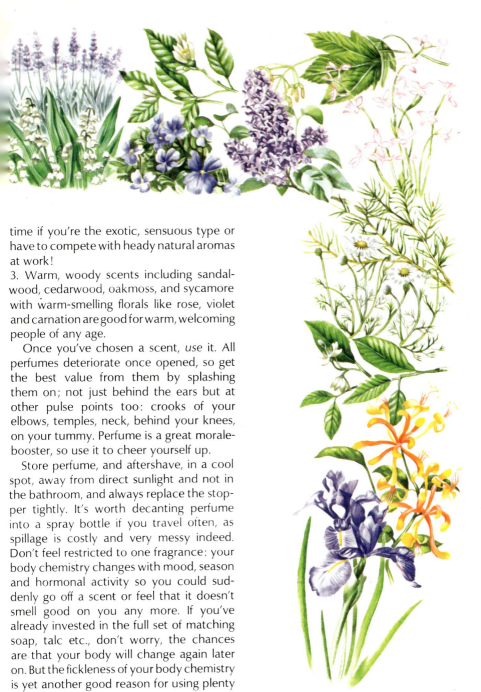

time if you're the exotic, sensuous type or have to compete with heady natural aromas at work!

3. Warm, woody scents including sandalwood, cedarwood, oakmoss, and sycamore with warm-smelling florals like rose, violet and carnation are good for warm, welcoming people of any age.

Once you've chosen a scent, *use* it. All perfumes deteriorate once opened, so get the best value from them by splashing them on; not just behind the ears but at other pulse points too: crooks of your elbows, temples, neck, behind your knees, on your tummy. Perfume is a great morale-booster, so use it to cheer yourself up.

Store perfume, and aftershave, in a cool spot, away from direct sunlight and not in the bathroom, and always replace the stopper tightly. It's worth decanting perfume into a spray bottle if you travel often, as spillage is costly and very messy indeed. Don't feel restricted to one fragrance: your body chemistry changes with mood, season and hormonal activity so you could suddenly go off a scent or feel that it doesn't smell good on you any more. If you've already invested in the full set of matching soap, talc etc., don't worry, the chances are that your body will change again later on. But the fickleness of your body chemistry is yet another good reason for using plenty of perfume, now!

# Recipes for health and beauty

Here are the underlined recipes from the diets on pp. 10-11. For every recipe there is a calorie count and a kilojoule count, its modern equivalent. The recipes can be used as part of the appropriate diet or as part of your own calorie or kilojoule-counted diet. They are good enough for the rest of the family to enjoy, and easy enough to prepare if you want to eat separately.

## BREAKFASTS

### Baked egg nest
1 medium egg, separated
pinch of salt
1 slice wholemeal bread

Whisk egg white with salt until stiff. Toast bread lightly. Pile egg white on toast and make a hollow in the centre. Slip the yolk into the hollow, and bake in a moderate oven or return to grill until yolk is set, white brown. Serves one.
Calories per serving: 147
Kilojoules per serving: 521

### Breakfast in a glass
1 egg
small carton natural yogurt
juice of 1 fresh orange or
2 tablespoons frozen orange
    juice, unsweetened
pinch of nutmeg

Whisk in blender or by hand, pour into a glass and serve immediately. Serves one.
Calories per serving: 163
Kilojoules per serving: 685

### Cottage eggs
4 eggs
4 tablespoons skimmed
    milk
knob of butter
200 gm (8 oz) cottage cheese

Beat eggs, milk and seasoning. Melt butter in non-stick saucepan, add egg mixture and cook gently. Add cottage cheese when mixture starts to set. Heat through. Serves four.
Calories per serving: 187
Kilojoules per serving: 784

### Devilled kidneys
400 gm (1 lb) lamb's kidneys
25 gm (1 oz) flour
1 finely chopped onion
0.25 litre ($\frac{1}{2}$ pint) skimmed
    milk
1 tablespoon Worcestershire
    sauce

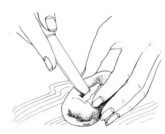

Skin and core kidneys, cut in half and toss in flour. Fry onion gently in a little oil for a few minutes, add kidneys. Stir in remaining flour, cook for a few seconds, then stir in milk and bring to the boil. Season, and simmer for five minutes. Serves four.
Calories per serving: 250
Kilojoules per serving: 820

## STARTERS

### Slimmers' tomato soup
1 chicken bouillon cube
0.25 litre ($\frac{1}{2}$ pint) boiling water
1 tablespoon chopped onion
200 gm (8 oz) can tomatoes
4 sticks celery
1 teaspoon Worcestershire
    sauce
seasoning

Put stock cube and water in a pan, add celery and onion and bring to the boil. Cover and simmer for 20 minutes until tender. Add tomatoes and sauce and simmer for 15 minutes. Strain or puree and season. Serves two.
Calories per serving: 25
Kilojoules per serving: 104

### Celery and tomato starter
4 sticks celery
25 gm (1 oz) cornflour
25 gm (1 oz) skimmed milk
    powder
100 gm (3$\frac{1}{2}$ oz) can pink
    salmon
6 large tomatoes
25 gm (1 oz) grated Edam
    cheese
chopped herbs

Cook chopped celery in water until tender. Blend cornflour with a little water until smooth, add skimmed milk powder, cel-